UNDERSTANDING THE

NURSING
PROCESS

THE NEXT GENERATION

NOTICE

Fifth Edition

UNDERSTANDING THE NURSING PROCESS

THE NEXT GENERATION

Mary Ellen Murray, Ph.D., R.N.

Director of Clinical Resources
Battle Creek Health System
Battle Creek, Michigan

Leslie D. Atkinson, R.N., M.S.N.

Nursing Program
Normandale Community College
Bloomington, Minnesota

Illustrated by Mark Atkinson

McGraw-Hill, Inc.

Health Professions Division

New York   St. Louis   San Francisco   Auckland   Bogotá   Caracas
Lisbon   London   Madrid   Mexico City   Milan   Montreal   New Delhi
Paris   San Juan   Singapore   Sydney   Tokyo   Toronto

Understanding The Nursing Process, Fifth Edition

Copyright © 1994 by McGraw-Hill, Inc. All rights reserved. Printed in the United States of America. Except as permitted under the United States Copyright Act of 1976, no part of this publication may be reproduced or distributed in any form or by any means, or stored in a data base or retrieval system, without the prior written permission of the publisher.

1234567890 DOCDOC 9876543

ISBN 0-07-105458-8

This book was set in Times Roman by University Graphics, Inc. The editors were Gail Gavert and Mariapaz Ramos -Englis; the production supervisor was Richard Ruzycka; the project was managed by Hockett Editorial Service; the text and cover were designed by Marsha Cohen, Parallelogram.
R. R. Donnelley & Sons was printer and binder.

Library of Congress Cataloging in Publication Data

Murray, Mary Ellen.
    Understanding the nursing process : the next generation / Mary Ellen Murray, Leslie D. Atkinson : illustrated by Mark Atkinson.—
5th ed.
        p. cm.
    Atkinson's name appears first on the earlier edition.
    Includes bibliographical references and index.
    ISBN 0-07-105458-8
    1. Nursing. 2. Nursing diagnosis. I. Atkinson, Leslie D.
II. Title.
[DNLM: 1. Nursing Process. WY 100 M9825a 1994]
RT41.A82   1994
610.73—dc20
DNLM/DLC
for Library of Congress   93-1938
                                                                CIP

This book is printed on acid-free paper.

Dedication
To Peter
To Erin and Derek

CONTENTS

CHAPTER FIVE

Implementation 113

CHAPTER SIX

Evaluation 123

PREFACE

Since the publication of the first edition of *Understanding the Nursing Process* in 1980, there have been major changes within the profession of nursing and within the health care system as a whole. The societal demand for quality health care and the necessity for cost containment have exerted pressure for a change in delivery systems.

In response to this dual pressure, nursing and medicine have collaborated to develop a health care delivery system that has proved effective in containing costs while simultaneously providing quality care. This system, *case management,* has been enthusiastically adopted by many hospitals. Still other hospitals have modified the system and experienced great success.

The nursing process has both stayed the same and changed in response to societal change. The constant aspect of the nursing process is the belief that the process is the way one "thinks as a nurse." This structured way of thinking has been a part of nursing as far back as the writings of Florence Nightingale!

The component of the nursing process that has changed is the *outcome* of the nursing process: the written plan of care. Thus, we have chosen to subtitle our text *The Next Generation.* By this subtitle we hope to recognize the contributions of nurse colleagues who have implemented the nursing process in another format: case management. Throughout the book we have discussed how the steps of the nursing process are incorporated into case management.

We continue to believe that the nursing process should be introduced in the first nursing course, even though students may not yet have the knowledge base to understand many aspects of care planning. Students continue to ask for a practical, understandable text on the nursing process, matched to their nursing level, as they begin to have clinical experiences. Since all "beginners begin at the beginning," this text is appropriate for use by students in all types of nursing programs. Because this text is written for a beginning student, terminology and nursing/medical interventions are presented only in the very practical sense of application to fundamental patient care situations.

This edition also incorporates the new American Nurses Association (ANA) Standards of Clinical Nursing Practice (1991) as well as the relevant nursing care standards from the Joint Commission on Accreditation of Health Care Organizations (AMH, 1992). Both of these documents reflect changes in the nursing process that emphasize documented outcomes and responses of the client to care.

Again, we wish to express and acknowledge our appreciation to colleagues and students (past and present) who have kept us honest throughout the first four editions. We congratulate NANDA members on the continued development of nursing diagnosis. We acknowledge the work of Gloria M. Bulechek, Ph.D., R.N., and Joanne C. McCloskey, Ph.D., R.N., and their research team at the University of Iowa for their contributions in defining and validating nursing interventions. Thank you also to Mark Atkinson for his cartoon art and to Tom Olson, Ph.D., R.N., University of Hawaii, for his initial work on Care Plan #2.

As always, the order of authorship of this text was determined by a flip of a coin and reflects our continued happy collaboration.

—MEM
—LDA

UNDERSTANDING THE
NURSING PROCESS
THE NEXT GENERATION

CHAPTER 1

Introduction to the Nursing Process

NURSING: WHAT IS IT?

Nursing has been described in many different ways by many different leaders and theorists in nursing. What is special about nursing? What service do we provide to our clients that no other health care professional provides? In 1980 the American Nurses Association, which is the professional organization for nurses in the United States, developed a definition that is current and basic to describe the scope of nursing practice.

> Nursing is the diagnosis and treatment of human responses to actual or potential health problems. (ANA, "Nursing—A Social Policy Statement," 1980)

This means, for example, that nursing is not responsible for diagnosing and treating cancer; the physician does this. Nursing is primarily responsible for diagnosing and treating a client's *response* to the cancer and medical treatment, such as inadequate nutrition, nausea, altered self-esteem, anxiety, and pain. Nursing is involved in aspects of the medical treatment as when giving a client prescribed medication or treatments, but the primary focus of nursing is the individual's response to health-related problems.

THE NURSING PROCESS: WHAT IS IT?

The nursing process is the way one thinks like a nurse. This process is the foundation, the essential, enduring skill that has characterized nursing from the beginning of the profession. Through the years the nursing process has changed and evolved, growing in clarity and understanding.

The nursing process is divided into five steps:

1. ASSESSMENT:
What brought you to the hospital?
Let me have a look at that.
Describe how you are feeling.

2. DIAGNOSIS:
What is the problem?
What is the cause?
How do I know it?

3. PLANNING:
What can I do about it?
What is most important?
What do I want to happen, by when?

4. IMPLEMENTATION:
Move into action.
Carry out the plan.

5. EVALUATION:
Did it work?
Why or why not?
Is the problem solved, or do I need to try again?

While these steps are an oversimplification, every nurse has already had much practice with the problem-solving or scientific process. Consider the college chemistry course that is required for all nurses. The students are asked to observe and examine the properties of different chemicals, and to perform a series of planned experiments utilizing those substances. Hopefully, the student, through the use of this scientific problem-solving process, has discovered the solution to the problem of how certain chemicals react. These steps are essentially the same as those used in the nursing process.

The nurse uses these five steps in *every* interaction with a client, no matter how brief a contact. Expert nurses have mastered this process to such a high degree that they are even unaware of using the separate steps in the process. In fact, in describing expert nursing practice, Benner states:

> It is not possible to recapture the explicit formal steps, the mental processes that go into experts' capacity to make rapid patient assessments. . . . To assume that it is possible to capture all the steps in nursing practice is to assume that nursing is procedural rather than holistic. Attempts may be made to model or make explicit all the steps that go into a nursing decision, but experts do not actually make decisions in this elemental, procedural way. They do not build up their conclusions, element by element; rather, they grasp the whole. Even when they try to give detailed accounts of the elements that went into their decisions, essential elements are left out. (Benner, 1984, pp. 42–43)

This process is the foundation, the essential, enduring skill that has characterized nursing from the beginning of the profession . . .

Assess: *"A careful nurse will keep a constant watch over her sick. . . . The feet and legs should be examined by the hand from time to time. . . ."*   *p. 17*

"For it may safely be said, not that the habit of ready and correct observation will by itself make us useful nurses, but that without it we shall be useless with all our devotion."   *p. 112*

Diagnose: *"I will tell you what was the cause of this hospital pyaemia being in that large private house. . . . It was that sewer from an ill-placed sink. . . ."*   *p. 30*

Plan: *"There are five essential points in securing the health of houses: pure air, pure water, efficient drainage, cleanliness, lights."*   *p. 24*

Implement: *"To be 'in charge' is certainly not only to carry out the proper measures but to see that everyone else does so too; to see that no one either wilfully or ignorantly thwarts or prevents such measures."*   *p. 42*

Evaluate: *"Surely you can learn at least to judge with the eye how much an oz. of food is, how much an oz. of liquid. You will find this helps your observation and memory very much. You will then say to yourself, 'A. took about an oz. of his meat today;' 'B. took three times in 24 hours about 1/4 pint of beef tea;' instead of saying, 'B. has taken nothing all day,' or 'I gave A. his dinner as usual.'*   *p. 113*

Adapted from: Florence Nightingale, *Notes on Nursing: What It Is and What It Is Not.* From an unabridged republication of the first American edition as published in 1860. (1969) New York: Dover Publications.

It is not that experts do not use the nursing process, but rather that they are so skilled in using it that it has become integrated into their thinking.

A more easily understood example of Benner's hypothesis is the skill of driving a car. Somewhere around age sixteen, most people (to the dismay and consternation of parental figures) begin a driver's education course. We all memorize and complete a driver's assessment before turning on the ignition:

first, walk around the car to check for obstacles and tire safety; then adjust mirrors, adjust driver seat height and distance from pedals, lock doors, adjust seat belt, check fuel gauge, and so forth. Finally, the driver can start the car and go! However, after a few years of experience, the driver just does these things automatically and probably would be unable to relate the steps that were so conscious only a short time ago. This book is to nursing what the driver's education manual is to driving!

One outcome of the use of the nursing process is a plan of care for the client. This plan of care may look very different from institution to institution. One hospital may choose a handwritten plan on a form devised for that purpose. Another hospital may use preprinted or computerized plans. But each of these contains the essential components of planned client care.

WHY IS THE NURSING PROCESS IMPORTANT?

Two driving forces have emerged in the 1990s that impact nursing practice: *emphasis on quality* and *emphasis on cost containment.* Nurses, like all health care providers, are responding to consumer demands for quality service. Nurses are continually seeking ways to improve their practice and the satisfaction of the clients they serve. If nursing is to survive the competitive challenges of the next decade, it must continue to provide a quality service that clients value. The nursing process provides a tool for the nurse to use in continually evaluating and improving the quality of nursing care. The second force is that of cost containment. Nurses have always been accountable for their professional practice, but now nurses are being required to accept financial accountability for their practice. This means that nurses need first to be aware of the resources used in caring for clients and then be in control of allocating the resources. Resources include not only supplies but the time nurses spend in providing care. Some decisions nurses are currently faced with include: Does this client need to be in the hospital, or can care be safely provided by a nurse visiting at home? Does this client have sufficient self-care knowledge to be discharged from the hospital? What teaching does this client need in order to have surgery on an outpatient basis? Both time and supplies have very real limits that will increasingly affect the decisions nurses make about care. The use of the nursing process helps to avoid duplications and omissions that result in the unnecessary use of resources.

The American Nurses Association, the organization of professional nurses in the United States, has published *Standards of Clinical Nursing Practice* (1991). Standards used in this sense define the responsibilities of all registered nurses engaged in clinical practice regardless of the setting (see Table 1-1). These standards list the nurse's responsibility to the public. The standards hold the nurse accountable for the use of the nursing process. It is important that students understand that the standards do not mandate that the use of the process must result in a specific form of care plan. That degree of specificity

TABLE 1-1   STANDARDS OF CLINICAL NURSING PRACTICE: STANDARDS OF CARE

Standard I.   **Assessment**
The Nurse Collects Client Health Data.

Standard II.   **Diagnosis**
The Nurse Analyzes the Assessment Data in Determining Diagnoses.

Standard III.   **Outcome Identification**
The Nurse Identifies Expected Outcomes Individualized to the Client.

Standard IV.   **Planning**
The Nurse Develops a Plan of Care that Prescribes Interventions to Attain Expected Outcomes.

Standard V.   **Implementation**
The Nurse Implements the Interventions Identified in the Plan of Care.

Standard VI.   **Evaluation**
The Nurse Evaluates the Client's Progress Toward Attainment of Outcomes.

Standards of Care in *Standards of Clinical Nursing Practice,* American Nurses Association, 1991. Used by permission.

is a function of the clinical setting in which the nurse is working. But the standards do require evidence of this critical thinking process, which all nurses use to plan and evaluate care.

In addition to meeting the Standards of Nursing Clinical Practice, there are other advantages to the nurse who becomes skilled in the use of the nursing process:

1.   *Graduation from an Accredited School of Nursing.*   All levels of nursing programs (diploma, associate degree, and baccalaureate) require students to have a basic competency in the use of the nursing process upon graduation.

2.   *Confidence.*   Care plans resulting from the nursing process let the student or the staff nurse know specifically what problems the client has, what goals are important for the client, and how and when they might best be accomplished.

3.   *Job Satisfaction.*   Good care plans can save time, energy, and the frustration that is generated by trial-and-error nursing from staff members and students whose efforts remain uncoordinated. Coordinating a client's nursing care through a care plan greatly increases the chances of achieving a successful resolution of health problems. The nurse and student should

feel a real sense of accomplishment and professional pride when outcomes in a care plan are met.

4. ***Professional Growth.***   Care plans provide an opportunity to share knowledge and experience. Collaboration with colleagues in formulating a nursing care plan will add to an inexperienced nurse's clinical skills. Later, during the process of evaluation, the nurse or student receives the feedback necessary to decide how effective the nursing care plan was in dealing with the client's problems. If the plan worked well, the nurse may use a similar approach in the future. If it failed, the nurse can explore possible reasons for the undesirable results with the client, other staff, other students, an instructor, or a clinical nurse specialist.

5. ***Aid in Staff Assignments.***   Care plans assist nurse managers, team leaders, and nursing instructors in making the most appropriate client assignments by showing the degree of complexity involved in an individual client's care plan. Could an aide follow the care plan and provide good care, or is a professional nurse required? Could students work with this client, or is the plan of care beyond their knowledge and experience? What aspects of nursing care can be safely delegated?

6. ***Employment in a Nationally Accredited Hospital.***   Hospitals are approved by a national commission to help ensure that clients receive quality care. The following statements are taken directly from the accreditation manual for hospitals and are a requirement for accreditation.

Nursing Process Components Required in Hospitals:
NC.1.3.4 The patient's medical record includes documentation of
   NC.1.3.4.1 the initial assessments and reassessments;
   NC.1.3.4.2 the nursing diagnoses and/or patient care needs;
   NC.1.3.4.3 the interventions identified to meet the patient's nursing care needs;
   NC.1.3.4.4 the nursing care provided;
   NC.1.3.4.5 the patient's response to, and the outcomes of, the care provided; and
   NC.1.3.4.6 the abilities of the patient and/or, as appropriate, his/her significant other(s) to manage continuing care needs after discharge.
NC.1.3.5 Nursing care data related to patient assessments, the nursing diagnoses and/or patient needs, nursing interventions, and patient outcomes are permanently integrated into the clinical information system (for example, the medical record).

There are also advantages for the client.

1. ***Participation in Own Care.***   If clients are able to help formulate their own care plans with the nurse, they gain a sense of their own ability to solve problems. When clients are active participants in their care, they are more likely to be committed to the outcomes in their care plans and thus achieve improved health.

2. ***Continuity of Care.***   The frustration of repeating the same information to each nurse caring for them is greatly reduced. Worries, concerns, and problems need not be communicated to each nurse to ensure that they are handled the way clients want them to be handled. The care plan communicates this information.

3. ***Improved Quality of Care.***   Use of the nursing process results in a thorough assessment of the client at the time of admission. Problems are identified at this time by an RN, who then develops a plan of nursing care with the client. This plan, developed by the nurse most familiar with the client, serves as a guide for other nurses, assistants, and students to follow in providing 24-hour care. Continuous evaluation and review of the plan of care assures a level of care that will better meet changing individual needs. This evaluation is a key part of the nursing process and a client's written care plan.

Giving nursing care without a care plan is like trying to cook a nameless entree without a recipe. To add to your troubles, you have to share the work for preparing this entree with three other cooks, all in the kitchen at different times. You can all cook, but a plan is needed to tell you what the entree is, how to prepare it, when to serve it, and how the three of you can coordinate your efforts to produce the best entree possible. Similarly, many nurses share in the care of a single client throughout the 24-hour hospital day. Each nurse is capable of providing care, but a plan is needed to coordinate their efforts.

NURSING PROCESS: THE NEXT GENERATION

The two major trends in health care in the 1990s, the demand for quality and the demand for cost containment, coupled with a cyclical nursing shortage have combined to encourage nursing leaders to seek new methods of delivering nursing care. One such system is the case management model, a delivery system in which the plan of both nursing and medical care is combined into one document, the case management plan, with the goal of providing quality care that is cost-effective. Zander has called case management plans "the second generation of nursing care plans," since they include both the nursing and medical diagnoses and specific time frames for achievement of outcomes (Zander, 1988).

In this system, physicians and expert nurses collaborate to develop a case management plan. This plan is a protocol for care of clients with a specific DRG (diagnosis related group). The plan lists the care and outcomes for each day of the expected hospitalization (Zander, 1988). An example might be a case management plan for a client with DRG 122: Uncomplicated Myocardial Infarction. Experienced nurses and physicians know that there are certain predictable problems that most clients with this diagnosis will develop. These professionals identify intermediate outcomes that are most likely to progress the client toward the discharge outcomes in a timely manner. Similarly, there are certain diagnostic procedures and medical treatments common to this medical diagnosis. Expert nurses can also predict that certain nursing diagnoses will have a high frequency occurrence. These nursing diagnoses are selected for the case management plan. Nursing experts have learned which nursing interventions are most likely to be effective in resolving the high frequency diagnoses, and these are the interventions selected for the plan.

In this system, the nurse is still accountable for assessment of the client, but the preprinted plan of care is designed to be appropriate for about 75% of the clients in a particular DRG category (Zander, 1988). The nurse is still accountable for adapting the plan for the individual client who may have additional problems or who may recover faster or slower than anticipated in the plan of care. Table 1-2 compares the steps of the nursing process to a case management plan.

TABLE 1-2   COMPARISON OF STEPS IN NURSING PROCESS VS. CASE MANAGEMENT PLAN

	Nursing Process	*Case Management Plan*
Assess	Individual client data	Pooled client data base
Diagnose	Individualized, based on nursing assessment	High frequency diagnoses from pooled data base of same DRG
Plan	Selected by one nurse based on one individual; timing independently selected by one nurse	Selected by multidisciplinary experts on time line
Implement	Focus on giving care	Focus on giving care
Evaluate	Document evaluation of client outcomes or progress toward outcomes	Document variance from expected outcomes, interventions, and time schedule

CHAPTER 2

Assessment

STANDARD I. ASSESSMENT

The Nurse Collects Client Health Data.

Standards of Care in *Standards of Clinical Nursing Practice*, American Nurses Association, 1991. Used by permission.

Assessment (data collection) is both the initial step in the nursing process and an ongoing component of every other step in the process. Assessment is a systematic, dynamic process by which the nurse, through interaction with the client, significant others, and health care providers, collects and analyzes data about the client (ANA, 1991). Assessment is part of each activity the nurse does for and with the client. The initial nursing assessment is the basis of the client care plan and later assessments contribute to revisions and updates in the plan as the client's condition changes. All individuals are constantly using their five senses to assess changes in their environment to make necessary changes and adapt to it. One person may note the cold temperature and dress more warmly while a second person is aware of a toothache and seeks dental care. Nurses too, are constantly seeking information about the client through their five senses and processing it to identify changes in status and intervene appropriately.

Assessing
   (Data   = Observation + Interview + Examination
Collection)

DATA COLLECTION

Initially the beginning nursing student collects data on the individual client, but families, groups, and communities can all be the focus of a nursing assessment by more advanced nurses. Even though the student may be focused on an individual client initially, it is essential that the student recognize the uniqueness of clients of different cultures. Often, nurses complete their assessment from the perspective of their own culture, with little consideration of the client's culture. What is considered "normal" in one culture may be unacceptable in another. As students become more experienced with assessment, family relationships and support systems, food preferences, communication styles, and health care beliefs are all included as aspects of client assessment.

Cultural Membership Influences Perception . . .

I had just returned to work as a staff nurse on the evening shift following an episode of what I had self-diagnosed as the flu. As the evening went on, my skin color began to change from white to a yellowish cast. This was alarming! After arranging for the care of my clients, I went down to the hospital emergency room to be evaluated. The young physician, an intern from Taiwan, began by noting my height and weight: 4' 11", 95 pounds. I also had long, dark, straight hair at that time. I told him that I was very concerned about my skin color. He responded, "You look fine to me!" "But this is not my normal color," I protested. As he noted the color of my sclera and ran further tests, he diagnosed hepatitis. We both had a good laugh over the incident and learned to evaluate assessment data from the perspective of the client's culture and racial origin.

Because human beings are extraordinarily complex and because assessment is an ongoing process, there is the potential for the nurse to collect an overwhelming amount of data. It is unrealistic to think that the nurse will record every bit of information that could be obtained. One component of the skill of assessment is the ability of the nurse to collect *relevant* data. The nursing care plan will be only as good as the data that go into it. A saying used by computerniks nicely illustrates this point, "Garbage in, garbage out."

Data Collection Format

Beginning nursing students are often required to complete nursing data collection assignments. Often these assignments are very lengthy and time-consuming. The purpose of such an assignment is to assist the student in a com-

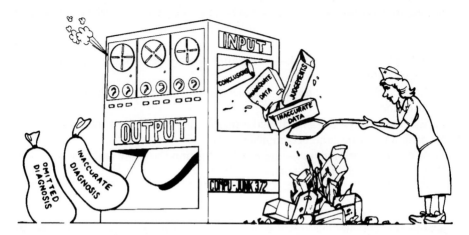

FIGURE 2-1.   Garbage in, garbage out.

prehensive data review and to avoid errors of omission. After the student has demonstrated proficiency in this skill, an abbreviated data collection format similar to those used by staff nurses is recommended. Several examples of such forms will be used throughout this book.

Most hospitals or other health care institutions use a form to guide the collection of data when the nurse is admitting the client. This form is usually labeled *Nursing Admission Assessment.* The structure of this form will vary with the institution. A structured form is used to avoid omitting data in important human response areas and to give the client an opportunity to discuss problems or request information in these areas. For example, when nurses (students and staff) complete an admission assessment, they frequently avoid initiating any discussion of sexuality or sexual behavior, either by skipping the item completely or by marking the item "NA," which means "not applicable." Although this may enhance the student's comfort level at the time, it does not contribute to a comprehensive assessment of the client. The nursing admission form includes this category thus identifying it as important and encouraging nurses to do more complete assessment even though there may initially be hesitancy or discomfort in asking questions in this area.

MASLOW'S BASIC NEED FRAMEWORK.   One assessment framework that is frequently used to guide the collection of data is based on the work of psychologist Abraham Maslow (1968), who postulated that all human beings have common basic needs that can be arranged in a hierarchical order (Table 2-1). Maslow further theorized that basic physical needs must be met to some degree before higher level needs can be met.

The basic physical needs such as food, fluid, and oxygen are considered survival needs and must be met, or at least partially met, if life is to continue. They are the lowest level of needs and are usually partially satisfied before

TABLE 2–1   COMMON BASIC HUMAN NEEDS

1. Physiological needs—needs that must be met, or at least partially met, for survival
2. Safety and security needs—things that make a person feel safe and comfortable
3. Love and belonging needs—the need to give and receive love and affection
4. Esteem needs—things that make people feel good about themselves; pride in abilities and accomplishments
5. Self-actualization needs—the need to continue to grow and change; working toward future goals

higher level needs. The nursing care of critically ill clients usually focuses on physiological needs. When the client improves, when life is no longer threatened, the satisfaction of higher level needs gains in importance. Higher level needs begin with safety/security needs and continue through self-actualization needs.

Using Maslow's theory of basic needs, consider the following data and their relationship to a basic need:

1.   PHYSIOLOGICAL NEEDS
—temperature 103°F
—respiration 36 per minute
—liquid stool four times in one hour
—complains of sharp continuous pain in right lower quadrant

2.   SAFETY–SECURITY NEED
—sleeps with night light
—"You won't forget me down in x-ray will you?"
—"Last time I was in the hospital I got my roommate's pill by accident."

3.   LOVE AND BELONGING
—parents are with Billy (hospitalized child)
—"We were married forty years when my wife died. I miss her so much."

4.   SELF-ESTEEM
—"I can't even control my bowels—just like a baby."
—"I can't go to physical therapy without a shower and a shave."

5.   SELF-ACTUALIZATION
—"My children are grown with families of their own. Raising them has been my biggest accomplishment."
—"Teaching nursing students is more than a job. I feel like I'm contributing to their development and to the profession."
—"There is so much to learn about caring for my baby."

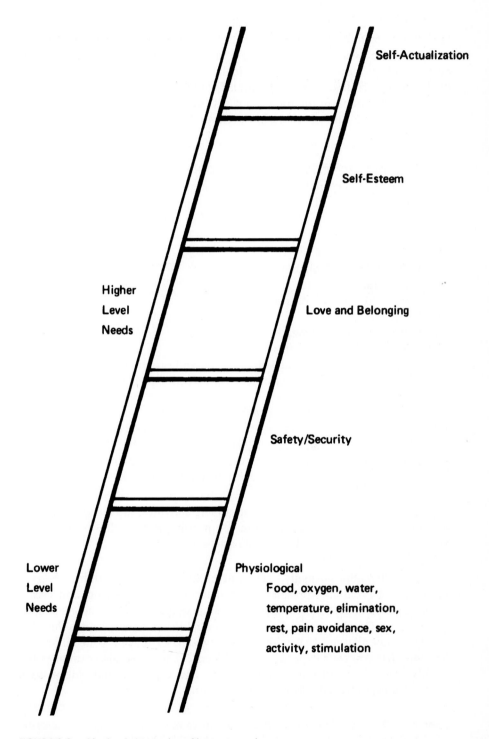

FIGURE 2-2.   Maslow's hierarchy of human needs.

The data recorded within each category may indicate the current status of need satisfaction, alterations in meeting the need, or perhaps interferences in meeting the need. By collecting data in each of these need categories, the nurse develops a format for systematically considering the total client rather than viewing an illness or a symptom. Comprehensive nursing care results from a consideration of the total client. At the end of this chapter there is an assessment form that uses Maslow's hierarchy of needs as an organizing framework.

HENDERSON'S COMPONENTS OF NURSING CARE.   Another framework which may be used to structure the nursing admission assessment was developed by nurse author Virginia Henderson. She described 14 needs or components of nursing care that a nurse may help the client to perform:

1. Breathe normally
2. Eat and drink adequately
3. Eliminate body waste
4. Move and maintain desirable posture
5. Sleep and rest
6. Select suitable clothing, dress and undress
7. Maintain body temperature
8. Keep the body clean and well groomed and protect the integument
9. Avoid dangers in the environment and avoid injuring others
10. Communicate with others
11. Worship according to one's faith
12. Work in such a way that there is a sense of accomplishment
13. Play, or participate in various forms of recreation
14. Learn, discover, or satisfy the curiosity that leads to "normal" development and health, and use available health facilities (Henderson, 1978)

After reading Henderson's list of nursing activities, the nurse can readily adapt the list to a data collection format. For example, the following questions and observations relate to Henderson's activities:

Activity 1. Breathe normally.   The nurse counts the respirations, observes the depth of breathing, presence of retractions or nasal flaring, and uses a stethoscope to listen for lung sounds. The nurse may also ask the client such questions as: Do you ever feel short of breath? What activity causes this? Do you have any allergies that make you congested or that make it difficult to breathe? Do you ever experience nosebleeds? The nurse also examines the nailbeds and extremities for color, warmth, and capillary refill. All of these observations indicate the level of oxygenation.

Activity 2. Eat and drink normally.   The nurse may ask the client to describe a normal day's diet, when the major meal of the day is taken, foods that cause the client problems, and to describe the resulting problems. The height, weight, and triceps skinfold may all be measured as a part of these data.

GORDON'S FUNCTIONAL HEALTH PATTERNS.   A third schema that is being used to structure nursing assessment is functional health pattern typology developed by Gordon (1982) (see Appendix A–Care Plan #1). Gordon proposes that the nurse assess the response pattern of the client in eleven areas and then evaluate to determine if the pattern is functional or dysfunctional for a particular client. The functional patterns specified by Gordon include:

1. Health Perception–Health Management Pattern
2. Nutritional-Metabolic Pattern
3. Elimination Pattern
4. Activity-Exercise Pattern
5. Sleep-Rest Pattern
6. Cognitive-Perceptual Pattern
7. Self-Perception–Self-Concept Pattern
8. Role-Relationship Pattern
9. Sexuality-Reproductive Pattern
10. Coping–Stress Tolerance Pattern
11. Value-Belief Pattern

NANDA'S HUMAN RESPONSE PATTERNS.   Another structure that may yield a future assessment format is the proposal by the North American Nursing Diagnosis Association (NANDA) (see Appendix A–Care Plan #2). This is an international group that has provided leadership in an effort to develop nursing diagnoses. The purpose of the organization is to develop, refine, and promote a taxonomy of nursing diagnostic terminology of general use to professional nurses (NANDA Bylaws: Article 1, Section 2) (Carroll-Johnson, 1991). Taxonomy here refers to an orderly classification of nursing diagnoses. NANDA proposes classifying nursing diagnoses using nine human response patterns (Taxonomy 1 Revised, June 1990): Exchanging, Communicating, Relating, Valuing, Choosing, Moving, Perceiving, Knowing, and Feeling. Nursing diagnoses are then organized under each of these patterns. With further development, this approach may yield a powerful assessment tool for nursing.

NURSING THEORIES.   The ultimate goal of nursing theory is to improve nursing practice. It is common for a school of nursing or a hospital to say that their nursing practice is based upon a certain nursing theory.

An example of such a practice might be the application of Orem's self-care deficit theory (1985). This nursing theory states that the client has health-related limitations in providing self-care. Thus it is the role of the nurse to assist the client in developing an optimal level of self-care. The nurse using this theory would focus on collecting data relative to self-care. For example, is the client able to have an adequate nutritional intake; is the client able to perform bowel and bladder elimination unassisted?

Another example of a nursing theory that could be used to guide assessment is the adaptation model of Sister Callista Roy (1984). Roy postulates that the client's coping activity is inadequate and it is the role of the nurse to promote the client's adaptive behaviors. The nurse practicing from this theory would focus on assessing the client's responses in each of four adaptive modes: physiology, self-concept, role function, and interdependence.

HUMAN GROWTH AND DEVELOPMENT.   Any format used for data collection is acceptable as long as it is thorough, comprehensive, and considers both the physiological and psychosocial aspects of the human being. In addition, any data collection approach must also include consideration of the individual's level of growth and development. Each chronological age has corresponding developmental tasks, both physical and psychosocial. A developmental task may be thought of as a job, a hurdle, a challenge, or an accomplishment related to a particular chronological age span. Illness may interfere with completion of developmental tasks appropriate to an age span or with progression to the next developmental level. During illness an individual may even regress to an earlier level of development. For example, the 3-year-old who has been toilet trained for 6 months may begin bed wetting again during hospitalization. The adolescent who has been menstruating for 6 months may cease to menstruate during a lengthy confinement in a body cast. Other individuals may appear to arrest at a developmental level during the stress of illness and hospitalization. For example, an infant may fail to begin to crawl and stand during illness. The infant may remain at the developmental level achieved prior to hospitalization and show very little new learning until the stress of hospitalization and illness is reduced.

Thus it is important for nurses to include assessment of developmental levels and tasks associated with each stage so they can recognize and understand variations from normal age-related development in clients. By recognizing that a child is regressing to an earlier level or is failing to keep up with peers' development, the nurse may be able to work with parents and other hospital staff to reduce the damaging influence that hospitalization is having on that child's development. The nurse who has a knowledge of developmental levels and the associated tasks will be able to further individualize nursing care. For example, adolescent developmental tasks focus on self-identity. While caring for adolescents, the nurse might choose a nonauthoritative approach that would allow the client the maximum amount of choice. Similarly, a school-aged child's developmental level focuses on independence and project completion. Nursing care that encourages the child's self-care will promote developmental growth. Table 2-2 is a brief summary of some of the major developmental tasks corresponding to chronological age.

Data Collection Skills

At the time the client is admitted to the hospital, the nurse begins planning nursing care for the client. This is begun using the skills of data collection.

TABLE 2-2   MAJOR DEVELOPMENTAL TASKS

1. Infancy—1 month to year
   —developing a sense of trust and belonging from relationship with mother and father
   —differentiating self from environment
   —learning to eat solid foods, to walk, to explore, to communicate
2. Toddler—1–3 years
   —developing will power, independence
   —learning to feed self, to run, communicate verbally, control elimination
   —exploring environment
3. Preschool—3–6 years
   —developing sexual identity
   —developing sense of initiative
   —working on autonomy, dressing self, washing
   —developing sense of time, space, distance
   —developing imagination
   —playing cooperatively
4. School age—6 to puberty
   —developing a sense of work; planning and carrying out projects
   —learning the skills for survival in the child's culture
   —developing modesty
   —learning to read, to calculate
   —developing neuromuscular coordination
   —learning to control emotions
5. Adolescent—12–20 years
   —developing physical maturity
   —developing autonomy from home and family
   —developing self-identity
   —coping with body image changes
   —identifying with peer group
6. Young adulthood—18–40 years
   —establishing enduring close physical and emotional relationships
   —child bearing, child rearing
   —establishing financial security
   —community responsibility
   —social interaction with peers
7. Middle adult—40–65 years of age
   —separating from children
   —establishing self in job
   —adapting to aged parents
   —adapting to physiological changes of aging
   —adjusting to altered relationship with spouse
8. Older adult
   —Accepting own life as valuable and appropriate

—Adapting to reduced physical health and strength
—Possible death of spouse
—Adjusting to retirement income
—Developing relationships with new family members
—Adapting to change in living location and style

Observation, interview, and examination are three methods the nurse uses to collect data. Although there are multiple sources the nurse may use for data collection, the client is always the primary source. Even if the client is unable to communicate verbally, the nurse can elicit valuable data using observation and examination skills. Additional data sources may be the client's past medical record (chart), significant others, and other persons giving care to the client. Professional journals, reference texts, and clinical nurse specialists are also important sources of data.

Nursing observations result in objective data. *Objective data* are factual data that are observed by the nurse and could be noted by any other skilled observer. During the assessment phase of the nursing process the nurse describes the signs or behaviors observed without drawing conclusions or making interpretations. At this point the nurse focuses on establishing a comprehensive data base about the client. Premature interpretation and analysis based on incomplete data may lead to errors. See Table 2-3 for examples of objective data. The column of judgments and conclusions demonstrates the interpretations of one individual nurse. Consider that "neatly groomed" may mean different things to different individuals and different cultures, whereas "hair combed, makeup applied" is concise and descriptive.

Contrasted with objective data are subjective data. *Subjective data* are information given verbally by the client. Examples of this type of data are the following statements:

"I feel so nervous."
"My stomach is burning."
"I want to be alone now."

From the examples of subjective data listed above each nurse could infer many different interpretations. For example, the nurse might guess that the client is nervous, fearing a diagnosis of cancer. This interpretation is not justified on the basis of the client's statement. The client could be nervous for many different reasons. The task during data collection is merely to observe, collect, and record data. Subjective data such as the examples in Table 2-4 are best recorded as direct quotes, thus providing the reader with the original information.

OBSERVATION.   Observation is a high level nursing skill that requires a great deal of practice. Consider a grocery shopping trip. Even though it is possible

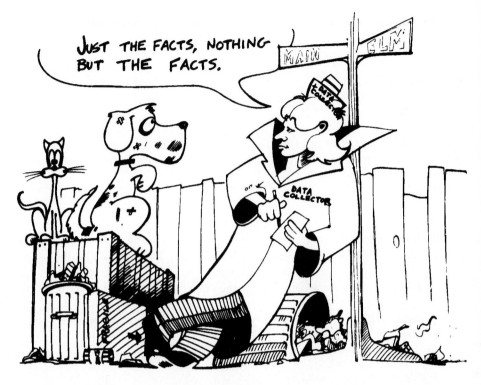

FIGURE 2-3.   The nurse records observations without drawing conclusions.

TABLE 2-3   OBJECTIVE DATA

Objective Data	Judgments and Conclusions
Hair combed, makeup applied	Improved body image
Drags right leg when walking	Intoxicated
Tremors of both hands	Client very afraid
250 cc dark amber urine	Voided large amount
Client in bed, covers over head, facing wall; no verbal response to questions	Client depressed
Administered own 8 A.M insulin using sterile technique	Understands self-administration of insulin
Ate cereal, juice, toast, coffee	Good appetite
Requests pain med q2h	Low pain tolerance

TABLE 2-4   SUBJECTIVE DATA

Subjective Data	Judgments and Conclusions
"Get out of my room."	Client is hostile
"I know something is wrong with my baby."	Client is anxious
"This catheter is killing me."	Client has pain
"Where am I? How did I get here?"	Client is confused
"I'm afraid they will find cancer when they operate."	Client worried about surgery

to have shopped at the store several times previously, few people can successfully recall all the items they need without a list or even find the location of all of the items they wish to purchase. The skills of observation and recall are difficult, but like all other skills they can be learned with systematic study and practice. The inexperienced student nurse will find it hard to perform nursing tasks and simultaneously continue the observation process. Yet it is

Observation is a high level nursing skill . . .

"What you want are facts, not opinions—for who can have any opinion of any value as to whether the patient is better or worse, excepting the constant medical attendant, or the really observing nurse? The most important practical lesson that can be given to nurses is to teach them what to observe–how to observe–what symptoms indicate improvement–what the reverse–which are of importance–which are of none–which are the evidence of neglect–and what kind of neglect."   *p. 105*

"But if you cannot get the habit of observation one way or other, you had better give up the being a nurse, for it is not your calling, however kind and anxious you may be."   *p. 113*

"In dwelling upon the importance of sound observation, it must never be lost sight of what observation is for. It is not for the sake of piling up miscellaneous information or curious facts, but for the sake of saving life and increasing health and comfort."   *p. 125*

Florence Nightingale, *Notes On Nursing: What It Is and What It Is Not.* From an unabridged republication of the first American edition as published in 1860. (1969) New York: Dover Publications.

this ability to perform constant, ongoing observation that is essential to assessment. For example, nursing students giving a first bedbath are concentrating so hard on the task that they may be unable to make observations or converse with the client. As students gain skill in giving physical care, they can shift their attention to the total client and begin to collect data through observation. They are now able to observe the skin condition, color, and temperature while bathing a client. The quality, depth, and effort of respirations can be noted. The ability of the client to move, as well as any pain associated with movement is noted. While giving a backrub, the skilled student can view the skin over the lower back, which is often an area of breakdown. The condition of the mucous membrane is noted during oral hygiene. The ability of the client to tolerate activity may also be observed as the nurse watches for signs of fatigue during and after the bath.

INTERVIEW.   The interview is a structured form of communication that the nurse uses to collect data. Both the ability to ask questions and the ability to listen are essential to successful interviews.

The nursing history or nursing admission assessment is one type of interview. This is completed by the nurse at the time of admission. The focus of the nursing history is the client's response to actual or potential health problems. As a part of this, the nurse reviews the client's past health history and coping methods that have been effective or ineffective. Data related to the client's life-style may also help to identify health risk factors. The nursing history is not a duplicate of the medical history, which has the disease process as its main focus. The purpose of the nursing history is to enable the nurse to plan nursing care for the client. The nurse clearly and directly conveys this purpose to the client at the beginning of the interview. The nurse may say something like, "Mr. Jones, I am Ms. Murray. I am the registered nurse who will be responsible for planning the nursing care you will receive while you are here. I would like to spend about a half hour with you now talking about your health history and completing this nursing admission form. This information will help me to work with you to begin to plan your nursing care." Note that the nurse has introduced herself in a professional manner and has clearly stated her professional accountability. If the institution uses them, this would be the appropriate time for the nurse to give the client a business card that also indicates a hospital telephone number where messages may be left when the nurse is not on the unit. This introduction is in contrast to, "Hi, I'm Anne and I'm your nurse. I need to ask you some questions."

Prior to beginning the nursing history, the nurse helps to make the client as comfortable as possible. This would include assessing for pain and doing what is necessary to reduce discomfort. It may also be helpful to offer the client the opportunity to go to the bathroom before beginning. Note that the nurse in the above example also gave the client some indication of the amount of time the interview would take. This is helpful to the client who may be expecting visitors or perhaps planning to make a telephone call. The nurse may also offer the client a beverage if medically permitted. This may help to

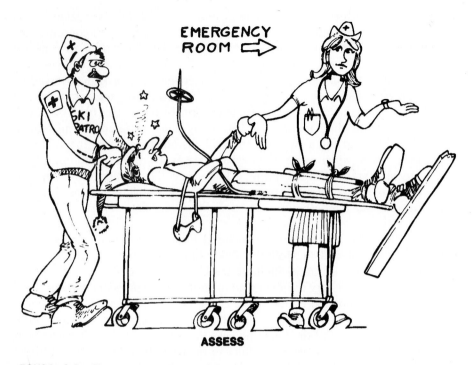

FIGURE 2-4. The nurse collects data through interviewing, observation, and examination.

put the client at ease and contribute to openness in the interview process. It is also helpful if the nurse sits during the interview at a level where eye contact between the nurse and the client can be easily maintained. This reduces the superior (nurse standing)-inferior (client in bed) feeling of the nurse-client relationship and conveys that the nurse has time to listen.

Most hospitals have a nursing history form that the nurse fills out on admission. This form guides or structures the interview, but the form is only a starting point. The nurse uses professional judgment to clarify areas of confusion or to elicit additional relevant data. The nurse does not form judgments or conclusions during the data collection phase, nor does the nurse rely on the judgments or conclusions of the client. For example the nurse does not ask the client, "Do you have problems with your bowel movements?" To this question the client may easily reply "No." This illustrates a judgment made by the client. Contrast this with the following dialogue between a nurse and a client:

NURSE: What is your normal pattern of bowel movements (BM)?
CLIENT: I have a BM about every other day.
NURSE: Has this changed since you broke your hip?
CLIENT: Yes—I feel constipated almost all the time.

TABLE 2-5   OPEN-ENDED QUESTIONS TO GUIDE ASSESSMENT OF HEALTH
PATTERNS

Focus	Nurse	Client Example
1. Normal pattern	"What do you usually eat for breakfast?"	"I like eggs and toast with lots of butter."
2. Effect of medical problems	"Has this changed since you've had this problem?"	"Yes, I really get heartburn from this."
3. Coping strategies	"Have you done anything different to help this?"	"Well, mostly I just skip breakfast or eat plain cereal. That helps."

NURSE: Have you done anything to treat your constipation?
CLIENT: Yes—I started to take a laxative both in the morning and in the evening. Sometimes it works too much and I get diarrhea, and other times I still feel constipated.

In this case the nurse has asked a series of open-ended questions (questions which may not be answered by yes or no) to assess the client's health pattern and has elicited a more comprehensive picture of the health pattern. The beginning nurse may wish to use the following series of questions to guide the assessment of each health area (Table 2-5).

1.   What is your normal pattern (or behavior)?
2.   Has your current health problem (illness, injury) affected your normal pattern (or behavior)?
3.   Have you done anything to help maintain or restore patterns (behavior) affected by your current health problem?

The nurse will probably find it helpful to take notes and actually complete most of the form during the interview process. Some explanation is always given to the client. The nurse may say, "Mr. Jones, I will be taking notes as we talk to make sure that I am accurate in recording this information." At the end of the interview it is helpful if the nurse summarizes the notes for the client, especially those areas where the current health problem has affected function or behavior. This contributes to the sense of trust in the nurse-client relationship and gives the client the opportunity to add or correct data.

Frequently, beginning nursing students are uncomfortable eliciting a nursing history. Students often state that they feel they are prying into personal matters. Students may be reassured that the client has the right to refuse to discuss any topic and that this right must be respected. When clients do choose to reveal personal data, nurses and students are responsible for assuring that the shared information remains confidential. Such data will remain within the context of the professional relationship and will be shared only with those who need the information to provide care.

The formal nursing interview is not primarily intended to be a treatment in and of itself, but is an organized format for data collection. Frequently, however, the client has a need to express feelings or share things that are worrisome and the nursing interview provides the opportunity and the uninterrupted attention of the nurse.

The informal aspect of the nursing interview is the conversation between

---

Often therapeutic communication may be the most appropriate skill to offer the patient . . .

I remember it as if it were yesterday—and it happened over 20 years ago! I was a third-year student nurse in a diploma program and I was working 3–11:30 P.M. on a rehabilitation unit. Most patients on this unit had survived a major trauma and were transferred to the unit for rehabilitation. Most of the patients were paraplegic or quadriplegic with little hope of return of function.

On this particular evening I had completed most of my work settling patients for the night. One young man, John, was very restless. He had been injured in a manufacturing accident and was permanently paralyzed from the waist down. He was very handsome, intelligent, and recently married at age 26 years. I had given him a muscle relaxant, a back rub, and assisted with hygiene. Though he usually retired early and slept soundly, tonight he seemed troubled and moody, not his usual self. At 11:10 I walked past his room and noticing his light still on, I entered his room to find him staring at the ceiling. "How's it going, John?" I asked as I settled into a chair at his bedside. "Do you want some company?" He invited me to stay and admitted he was at "rock bottom." We talked a long time and in the conversation that followed he revealed that he and his wife had always wanted children, and that there was still the chance that physically he could father a child. "But," he confided, "what would a kid think of having a father in a wheelchair?"

I told him! For my father had multiple sclerosis and had suffered a progressively degenerative course to where he was ultimately a quadriplegic. I told him of the tough times, of the things I missed or envied in my friends' fathers, but I told him too of the love and support of my father . . . of the closeness of our relationship . . . of my respect for and pride in my father. "But," John said, "that was because you were a girl. What if I had a son?" I couldn't answer for my brother, I said, but I could describe my family life. After a long time, John said, "Thank you, you've helped." I finished my charting and when I left the unit his light was out and he was sleeping.

the nurse and the client in the course of giving nursing care. The close relationship developed while the nurse is giving physical care frequently enables the client to express concerns. The nurse who can skillfully give physical care is then free to simultaneously focus attention on what the client is saying.

The planned, deliberate communication the nurse uses to help identify and meet the health care needs of the client is called *therapeutic communication*. Like other nursing skills, therapeutic communication requires practice to be effective. It may be difficult for beginning nursing students to give physical care while simultaneously engaging in therapeutic communication. Often, for example, the nurse uses the time spent giving a bedbath as an opportunity for therapeutic communication. This is often an unhurried, private time for conversation between the nurse and the client. With practice the nurse is able to focus on what the client is saying. During this communication the nurse also continues to make observations.

At other times, the nurse will plan a period of time for the sole purpose of engaging in therapeutic communication. This, too, may be difficult for the beginning student who may feel uncomfortable approaching clients without a technical skill (such as taking a blood pressure) to "do for" the client. Often therapeutic communication may be the most appropriate skill to offer the client. This may be the case when a client is afraid, discouraged, or has just been told of a serious diagnosis.

EXAMINATION.   The final activity of data collection is examination. A complete physical examination is a skill beyond the scope of most registered nurses and is usually done by nurses with advanced education and training. A partial physical examination that is limited to an area of practice or that focuses on a specific problem is an expected skill of all nurses. Before beginning the physical process of examination, the nurse establishes a relationship with the client. The nurse always precedes the examination with an explanation of the procedure and requests the client's permission to proceed. The nurse always provides for the client's privacy, closing doors and pulling curtains as necessary. The nurse checks with clients and asks if they would prefer if their visitors wait outside the room before beginning. The nurse might say something like, "Mrs. Jones, I'd like to do a physical examination now with your permission. If you feel any discomfort will you please tell me? I'll begin by checking your eyes and ears." When doing only a partial physical examination, the nurse might state, "I'd like to take a look at your stitches and the drain site to make sure everything is healing."

The nurse is then ready to begin a physical examination of the client. The nurse may choose to conduct a total body assessment or to focus on one or more specific areas such as lung sounds, stitches, or a wound or a drain. If a client complains of a generalized pain, the nurse may conduct a very thorough examination. In contrast, if a child in the emergency room fell from a bicycle and shows the nurse a large bleeding laceration on the elbow, this might be the initial focus of the examination. It is important that the nurse conducts a thorough examination as soon as possible since internal injuries that are not so readily apparent may also be present.

In obtaining this examination data, the nurse uses a systematic approach to avoid omissions. For nursing students, the particular curriculum of a school may require a certain approach. Hospitals may, by the forms they provide, structure the examination done by a practicing nurse. It really does not matter which approach is used as long as it is methodical and the nurse uses it consistently to gain a high degree of skill. One nurse may follow a *cephalocaudal* (head to toe) approach, which begins with an assessment of the hair, skull, eyes, ears, nose, mouth, and facial skin and moves in a downward direction. Another nurse may select a *body system* approach, which may begin with a consideration of the respiratory system, moving to the digestive system, to the cardiovascular system and so forth. Any methodical, thorough approach is acceptable as long as it meets the need to gather relevant data that help to identify health problems requiring nursing intervention.

During physical examination, the nurse uses senses and skills to gather information about the client. *Visualization* is inspection of the client's body. This is coupled with the use of the senses such as hearing, smelling (certain disease processes or physical changes are associated with characteristic odors), and touching. Visualization is often the most appropriate starting place for a physical examination because the nurse will not cause the client any discomfort. The nurse also uses the skill of *auscultation*, which includes listening with a stethoscope to heart, lung, and bowel sounds. Next the nurse may palpate or feel the body. This may give the nurse information about organ position, body temperature, abnormal growths, abdominal rigidity, or the location of pain. Some nurses may be skilled in the use of *percussion*, the tapping of a body surface with a rubber-tipped mallet or with the fingers. This is done to elicit responses, usually in the form of sound or movement, that give information about an underlying body part. For example, it is common practice to percuss a distended abdomen for a drumlike sound indicating retained flatus (gas) in the bowel following abdominal surgical procedure.

While it is necessary to establish a relationship with the client prior to examination, the examination itself can be a tool for showing concern and enhancing the relationship. The nurse who stops to palpate the abdomen and listen to bowel sounds when the client complains of pain shows concern for the client, identifies possible changes in client status, and establishes credibility. The observations the nurse makes during the examination are recorded as objective data: 3-inch scar, left lower quadrant; temperature 98.6°F; blood pressure (BP) 110/70; no bowel sounds present.

During the assessment phase the nurse has the potential to collect volumes of data about a client. Throughout the process it is important to consider the significance of the data to the task at hand, which is identifying problems and planning nursing intervention. As the student practices data collection, skill is gained in eliciting and recording relevant data. It is also essential that the student learns to report data in a timely manner to the appropriate person. If the physician sees the client once a day, and a major change in he client's condition is noted after that visit, it is the responsibility of the nurse to report this immediately in addition to completing the necessary documentation.

ASSESSMENT: THE NEXT GENERATION

A nurse who is caring for clients in a hospital where a case management model is used to deliver nursing care will experience a different, but no less important, need for assessment skills. In this setting, a client is admitted to the hospital with a medical diagnosis made by the physician. This diagnosis corresponds to a certain DRG (diagnosis related group) that specifies the usual length of hospital stay for a client. Expert nurse clinicians who have cared for many clients with that specific medical diagnosis and DRG have worked collaboratively with physicians to determine a case management plan combining both nursing care and medical care. These expert nurses, based on their experience, know what are the usual or customary problems associated with a given medical diagnosis. The nurse admitting the client completes the initial assessment as described above. The nurse then uses the assessment to determine that the case management plan is appropriate for this particular client and to individualize the plan.

Another example may help to make this clear. From a knowledge of growth and development, nurses know that most children are walking by 2 years of age. If the nurse is providing care for a child who is 2 1/2 years old and who is not walking, this is a deviation from what is expected. The nurse observes this on the initial assessment. A care plan that assumes the mobility of the average 2-year-old may need to be modified for this child. So it is with the use of a case management plan of care. It may correctly be assumed to "fit" the vast majority of clients. In fact, it is estimated that a case management plan identifies outcomes and guidelines for managing approximately 75% of clients in a particular DRG category (McKenzie, 1989). However, the nurse still has the responsibility to assess the client and to validate as necessary.

SUMMARY

Assessment is the first step in the nursing process and the one step that is a part of every other step in the nursing process. The nursing assessment that the nurse completes upon the client's admission to the hospital is focused on the client's response to actual or potential health problems. During assessment the nurse collects data by interview, observation, and examination. The nurse does not make judgments or conclusions at this time but focuses on establishing a comprehensive data base that reflects the health status of the client. Similarly the nurse seeks to gather only data, not judgments and conclusions, from the client by the use of open questions: "What is your normal pattern of . . . ? Has it changed with illness? Are you doing anything to cope with the changes?"

PRACTICE EXERCISE

I. Consider the following pieces of data and label them:
O = objective
S = subjective
J = judgment or conclusions.

1. 75 cc dark amber urine.
2. Client is afraid of surgery because her mother died in the hospital.
3. "I can't go that long (8 hours) without smoking."
4. Large amount bright red drainage from incision site.
5. Client states that the pain is 8 on 1–10 scale.
6. Respiratory rate of 36 after walking length of hall unassisted.
7. Client's oral intake is in excess of body requirements.
8. Intelligent and articulate middle-aged adult.
9. Confused elderly white male.
10. Client is becoming increasingly agitated.

II. Given the following client responses, formulate two additional questions the nurse might ask that would encourage the client to provide more complete information about his or her response to actual or high-risk health problems.

1. Client is 86-year-old woman with arthritis, living alone in own home. You are to assess her mobility status.
   NURSE: "Do you have any problems getting around?"
   CLIENT: "Nope."
2. Client is 12-year-old boy with possible appendicitis. You are to assess pain.
   NURSE: "Are you having any pain?"
   CLIENT: "No—can I go home now?"
3. Client is 45-year-old woman, slightly overweight. You are to assess the client's nutritional status.
   NURSE: "Do you have any nutritional problems?"
   CLIENT: "None other than eating too much."
4. Client is 53-year-old man admitted for possible heart attack. You are to assess the client's coping skills/stress management.
   NURSE: "Do you feel that you are under a lot stress?"
   Client: "No more than most people."
5. Client is 17-year-old high school football team captain admitted for diagnostic tests possibly for mononucleosis. You are initiating the nursing assessment.
   NURSE: "How have you been feeling?"
   CLIENT: "Not too bad."

ANSWERS TO EXERCISE ON ASSESSMENT

I.

1.	O	**6.**	O
2.	J	**7.**	J
3.	S	**8.**	J
4.	J (Use of word "large" makes it a judgment.)	**9.**	J (Describe the behaviors that made you label the client as confused. State the client's age.)
5.	S	**10.**	J (Describe the behaviors that made you label the client as agitated.)

II.

1. "Can you tell me how you manage things—like cooking and grocery shopping?"
   "Has your arthritis made this hard for you to do?"
   "What things have you figured out that help you?"
2. "It sounds like you want to get out of here. Have you ever been in a hospital before?"
   "What was that like for you?"
   "What did the nurses do then that helped you?"
   "Do you think that if your side stops hurting you can go home?"
3. "What would be a typical breakfast, lunch, supper for you?"
   "What do you like for snacks?"
   "Are you able to exercise?"
4. "How much stress is normal for 'most people'?"
   "How do you cope with stress?"
   "Does it work for you?"
5. "What is 'not too bad' for you?"
   "And what do you do when you feel like that?"
   "Does that help?"
   "What problems brought you into the hospital or to the doctor?"

CASE STUDY: DATA COLLECTION

The case study method will be used throughout this book to illustrate the steps of the nursing process. The same case study of Mrs. Witten will be found in each chapter to illustrate the various steps in the nursing process. The following pages illustrate the nursing assessment that was done for Mrs. Witten upon admission.

89714530
Witten, Laura
6/3/94 room 511
Dr. Ronal/Keller

NURSING ASSESSMENT

(Data Collection Format based on Maslow's basic needs framework)

General Information

Information given by: client

Name: Mrs. Laura Witten

Age: 45 years   Sex: female   Race: Caucasian

Admission date/time: 6/3/94; 9 A.M.

Admitting medical diagnosis: Possible Cholecystitis/Cholelithiasis

Arrived on unit by: wheelchair   from: home

Accompanied by: husband

Admitting weight/VS: T. 99.0, P. 96, R. 28, BP 138/88; 148 lbs, 5'4"

Client's perception of reason for admission: severe pain in right upper quadrant; "It has never been this bad before. I couldn't stand it at home. The doctor thinks it might be my gallbladder"

How has problem been managed by client at home? "I took 2 aspirins but that just didn't help at all; it made me nauseated"

Allergies: no known allergies

Medications: ASA 10 gr for pain in abdomen; no prescription meds

Physiological Needs

OXYGENATION: Some restlessness, R. 28, reports no difficulty breathing; states nonsmoker; clear breath sounds; no cough; P. 96, strong and regular; no murmurs heard, denies any chest pain; 2–3 second capillary refill of fingernail beds; no ankle or leg edema; skin pink but pale

TEMPERATURE MAINTENANCE: T. 99.0; denies a fever in the last few days; states she feels warm now

NUTRITIONAL–FLUID: 5′4″, 148 lbs; states she has gained about 20 lbs over the last 5 years; states she has been eating regular meals (3 meals a day and occasional nighttime snack) and not dieting; reports food sometimes helps the discomfort; reports greasy or rich, buttery foods make her sick (nausea & vomiting); good skin turgor; has not eaten for 10 hours but has taken fluids; last intake 1 hour ago—large glass of gingerale and ice that she sipped and kept down; slight nausea now

ELIMINATION: last bowel movement 6/3; normal pattern qod; denies stool hard or difficult to pass; denies any problem with urination; states normal large amounts every few hours, no burning

REST–SLEEP: usually retires at 10:30 P.M. and sleeps until 7 A.M.; states no problem sleeping at home but has never been in hospital and "with this pain I was not able to sleep much last night"; denies use of sleeping pills

PAIN AVOIDANCE: rates pain as an "8" on a 1–10 scale; says it started last night and has gotten worse; it is a continuous sharp pain in right upper quadrant; reports a few previous attacks over the last year that have lasted a few hours and then subsided; clenching hands and gritting teeth; restless

SEXUALITY–REPRODUCTIVE: last menstrual period 5/20; states she is fairly regular on a 28–30 day cycle; denies use of any birth control, states husband had a vasectomy after the birth of their third child 7 years ago; denies any concerns with sexual aspect of her life or role as a woman

STIMULATION–ACTIVITY: states she is active and has no problems; states she walks around the block occasionally; works part-time as a clerk in a children's store; enjoys TV

Safety–Security Needs

She is oriented and alert; responds appropriately to questions; states she wears glasses and really needs them; states she is "scared of being in the hospital and of being sick" and has never been in the hospital other than for the birth of her children; tears in eyes; diaphoretic, hands trembling; last PAP test was 2 years ago and negative; last breast exam 2 years ago, states she was never really taught breast self-exam and does not do it; husband here and plans to stay with her

Love–Belonging Needs

has 3 children; husband with her

Self-Esteem Needs

"I'm never sick; the doctor thinks it might be my gallbladder causing all the trouble. I don't mean to act like a baby but this pain is so bad; I was supposed to work today and the kids will be worried about me when they get home from school but Bob (husband) will be there today for them. They really count on me being there when they get home. 'MOM' is the first thing they holler when they come through the door after school"

Self-Actualization Needs

(No data.)

CHAPTER 3

Diagnosis

STANDARD II. DIAGNOSIS

The Nurse Analyzes the Assessment Data in Determining Diagnoses.

Standards of Care in *Standards of Clinical Nursing Practice*, American Nurses Association, 1991. Used by permission.

Diagnosis is the second step in the nursing process and is the phase during which the nurse analyzes the data gathered during assessment and identifies problem areas for the client. The nurse then makes a nursing diagnosis. The terms *nursing diagnosis* and *diagnosing* do not mean the same thing in this chapter and may be confusing for the student. *Diagnosing* is a process of data analysis and problem identification. It is a form of decision making that the nurse uses to arrive at judgments and conclusions about clients' responses to actual or potential health problems. A *nursing diagnosis* is the specific result of diagnosing and is the problem statement that nurses use to communicate professionally. It refers to a problem statement that the nurse makes regarding a client's condition. The American Nurses Association defines nursing diagnosis as a clinical judgment about the client's response to actual or potential health conditions or needs (1991). It is helpful to think of these terms as a noun (nursing diagnosis) or verb (diagnose) to distinguish between the two.

There are three activities in the diagnosis step:

Diagnosing = Data Analysis + Problem Identification + Formulation of Nursing Diagnosis

---

DATA ANALYSIS

QUESTION: "So now that I've got all these data, what do I do with them?"
ANSWER: "Make sense out of them and use them."

The nurse has completed the initial systematic data collection and is now ready to begin the process of analysis. The nurse begins the activity of data analysis by considering all the data that were gathered during the assessment phase of the nursing process. The nurse quickly checks for completeness of the data. For example, if the data were collected in a format that used Maslow's hierarchy of basic needs, it may be that data about rest and sleep patterns were unclear, incomplete, or omitted. The nurse may decide to go back and gather additional data as needed.

Another aspect of completeness is the cultural context of the data. While it may be difficult for nurses to go beyond the perspective of their own cultures, it is essential to analyze the data within the context of the culture of the client. An example of this is a consideration of how pain is expressed within various cultures. Some cultures are open in expressing pain, while others place a high value on stoicism and self-control. It is necessary for the nurse to be sensitive to the culture of the client and to assure that data collection includes the client's cultural uniqueness.

The nurse also looks for inconsistencies or ambiguity in the data. It may become apparent to the nurse that the sequence of events in the history is contradictory and needs to be resolved. Two data sources may also be inconsistent. For example, the client may report having only an occasional "social drink," while the spouse gives data about "drinking 10–12 cans of beer daily." At this point no judgment is made about the existence of a problem, but the inconsistency is noted. Another example might be that the nurse does not understand from reading the assessment what methods the client has used for pain relief and with what result.

The data are evaluated for comprehensiveness—do the data give a complete picture of the client, considering both physical and psychosocial aspects of the person? The nurse asks whether the assessment has considered all areas that may be relevant to the client. This considers such things as higher level needs, cultural factors, data related to growth and development, in addition to the more obvious physical areas. These factors taken all together comprise holistic health—that is, the concept that the mind and the body are inseparable and one cannot be treated without the other. In summary, the nurse reviews the data for clarity, consistency, completeness, and comprehensiveness.

After reviewing the data the nurse is ready to begin analysis. This is the process of studying the data and making judgments and conclusions about the meaning of the data. The nurse will decide if the data indicate a problem for the client or a situation which puts the client at risk for the development of problems in the future. The following decisions are made based on the data:

1. Determine whether measurement data are within the normal range for the client and within the norms for that client's age group. For example, if the nurse has taken the blood pressure of the client, the nurse can now ask if this pressure is typical for this individual. The nurse also determines if this BP reading is within the normal range for this client's age.

2. Determine if functioning described by the client is typical of past functioning and within normal patterns for the client's age. The nurse could consider the bowel elimination pattern that the client reported as "every other day, soft and easy to pass, no blood, no use of laxatives but daily bran flakes, no change with diabetes" and decide that the pattern is both typical for the client and within normal patterns for adults.

3. Determine what relationships exist between pieces of data. For example, if the data reveal that the client is 25% overweight, has an elevated blood pressure, and has no understanding of caloric content of food and body requirements, the nurse recognizes the relationship between the many factors affecting the obesity. Another client may be unable to sleep, appear very anxious, be very demanding of the nurses' time, and have a history that includes a parent who died during a routine surgical procedure. While the obvious interpretation that the client is also worried about dying during surgery needs confirmation by the client, it seems clear that there is a relationship between the data.

4. Evaluate the physical assessment data as positive, negative, normal, or abnormal signs or findings. For example, if the nurse has completed auscultation of the client's lungs, the nurse makes a decision if the findings were normal or not; and if not, which abnormality was heard and the location of the abnormal sound. This is clearly recorded. Similarly the decision that a particular aspect of the examination was negative is valuable because it notes that a judgment has been made and a problem ruled out. These decisions may be difficult for the beginning nurse to make. Until the nurse has had a lot of experience, it is difficult to judge what are normal versus what are abnormal lung sounds. The student should not hesitate to ask a more experienced nurse to assist in this evaluation.

5. Determine whether specific behavior patterns contribute to the health and well-being of the client. The nurse may evaluate that dietary and exercise patterns of the client foster cardiovascular health as in the case of the client who reports that she has never smoked, has decreased her intake of red meat to twice a week, and walks two miles a day several times a week. The nurse considers the opposite decision in the case of the client who reports that she is a pack a day smoker, "my father died of a heart attack," needs to lose 30 pounds, and has no physical activity. Here the nurse would also try to determine if the client perceives these things to be problematic and if the client is willing to make any life-style changes. While the nurse may evaluate something to be a problem, the adult client always has the right to make a decision to refuse the health professional's recommendations. Although this may generate feelings of ineffectiveness and frus-

tration in the nurse, it is the goal of health education to assist clients in making informed decisions, and it is the right of clients to make decisions within the context of their own values, beliefs, and culture.

6. Determine the strengths and resources, as well as limitations, of the client as they affect health status. These may include such things as cognitive abilities or potential, willingness to change, family support, economic resources, and available time to invest. For example, a nursing student who is going to school full-time and working part-time would probably have little time, energy, or money to invest in an exercise club. For another client, the nurse may make the judgment that the YMCA membership the client holds is a valuable resource affecting health status. Another client who has suffered a mild heart attack may state, "That was a warning. Now I am ready to do whatever I have to, to get healthy and stay healthy." The nurse may interpret that as a willingness to receive health teaching and a motivation to follow through.

PROBLEM IDENTIFICATION

The next step is to identify a broad focus area requiring nursing intervention, such as nutrition, elimination, or incorrect or inadequate information. This is the identification of a problem area. Nurses use both nursing theory, general knowledge base, and cumulative experience to define this area. For example, in a client who is a newly diagnosed non–insulin dependent diabetic, the nurse may read data that include such things as: a history of being overweight since childhood, "My mother used to bake me a chocolate whipped cream cake if I got a good report card," "I've tried every diet in the book," "I don't feel jolly—aren't fat people supposed to be jolly?" "My children are plump but it is just baby fat and they'll grow out of it," client is 43 years old, 5'2", weight 189 lbs. The nurse uses a knowledge of human growth and development, behavioral psychology, anatomy and physiology, and nursing in considering these data. A focus for nursing intervention in the area of nutrition is indicated.

In a second example, another client may include the following data: pain in the lower back, unable to perform job (cashier in grocery store) because it causes pain, unable to do any housework without aggravation of pain, "I'm no use to anybody," "My mother had a bad back and she was an invalid at age 45." Here the nurse also uses the knowledge of sciences related to nursing to recognize that the data indicate an area for nursing intervention. The nurse identifies the back pain as the most immediate problem focus area requiring intervention, although there are data to indicate that the client is also experiencing low self-esteem.

After a broad focus area is chosen, a narrower, more specific problem statement is selected from the diagnostic statements developed by NANDA.

> **NURSING DIAGNOSIS:**
> *is a clinical judgment about the client's response to actual or potential health conditions or needs. (ANA, 1991)*

At this point the student may choose to consult the *Nursing Diagnosis Pocketbook* that is included with this text. Table 3-1 lists the problem focus areas corresponding to basic human needs. Specific nursing diagnoses developed by NANDA are listed under each focus area. Alternatively, the student may use Table 3-2, which is an alphabetized listing of NANDA diagnostic categories. These are organized according to nine human response patterns as a broad focus area.

The next step in the process is to move from the completed data analysis with the identification of a focus area to the determination of the correct nursing diagnosis. Consider the following data that the nurse has documented from the admission nursing history of the client Mrs. Jones:

—54 years old, has had three children
—complains of involuntary loss of urine "when I cough or sneeze or in exercise"
—"I have to go to the bathroom all the time—I can't sit through a movie without having to get up to use the restroom."

The nurse reviews the basic needs framework of Maslow and selects a focus area of *Elimination Needs*. Further review of the two major categories in this area indicates a choice between *Bowel* or *Urinary* elimination, and the nurse selects the subcategory of *Urinary Elimination*. Nursing diagnoses under this category include:

* Functional incontinence
* Reflex incontinence
* Stress incontinence
* Toileting self-care deficit
* Total incontinence
* Urge incontinence
* Urinary retention

The nurse can easily eliminate two diagnoses: toileting self-care deficit, and urinary retention. Neither of these is related to the symptoms that the client has evidenced. Now the nurse uses a process of matching the client's symptoms to the defining characteristics of the nursing diagnoses. For example, the nursing diagnosis of reflex incontinence has as defining characteristics: no awareness of bladder filling; no urge to void or feelings of bladder fullness.

TABLE 3-1   NURSING DIAGNOSES ORGANIZED BY BASIC HUMAN NEED

1. **Oxygen Needs**
   —Altered (specify type) tissue perfusion (renal, cerebral, cardiopulmonary, gastrointestinal, peripheral)
   —Decreased cardiac output
   —Dysfunctional ventilatory weaning response
   —High risk peripheral neurovascular dysfunction
   —Impaired gas exchange
   —Inability to sustain spontaneous ventilation
   —Ineffective airway clearance
   —Ineffective breathing pattern
   —High risk for aspiration
   —High risk for suffocation
2. **Temperature Maintenance**
   —Ineffective thermoregulation
   —Hypothermia
   —Hyperthermia
   —High risk for altered body temperature
3. **Nutritional and Fluid Needs**
   —Altered nutrition: less than body requirements
   —Altered nutrition: more than body requirements
   —Altered nutrition: potential for more than body requirements
   —Effective breastfeeding
   —Feeding self-care deficit
   —Fluid volume deficit
   —Fluid volume excess
   —High risk for fluid volume deficit
   —Ineffective breastfeeding
   —Ineffective infant feeding pattern
   —Interrupted breastfeeding
   —Impaired swallowing
4. **Elimination Needs**
   Bowel:
   —Bowel incontinence
   —Constipation
   —Colonic constipation
   —Diarrhea
   —Perceived constipation
   Urinary:
   —Altered urinary elimination
   —Functional incontinence
   —Reflex incontinence
   —Stress incontinence
   —Toileting self-care deficit
   —Total incontinence

—Urge incontinence
—Urinary retention
5. **Rest and Sleep Needs**
   —Fatigue
   —Sleep pattern disturbance
6. **The Need for Pain Avoidance**
   —Pain
   —Chronic pain
7. **Sexual Needs**
   —Altered sexuality patterns
   —Sexual dysfunction
8. **Stimulation Needs**
   —Activity intolerance
   —Diversional activity deficit
   —Impaired physical mobility
   —High risk for activity intolerance
   —High risk for disuse syndrome
   —Sensory/perceptual alterations (specify: visual, auditory, kinesthetic, gustatory, tactile, olfactory)
   —Unilateral neglect
9. **Safety and Security Needs**
   Physiological level:
   —Altered health maintenance
   —Altered oral mucous membrane
   —Altered protection
   —Dysreflexia
   —Impaired home maintenance management
   —Impaired skin integrity
   —Impaired tissue integrity
   —High risk for impaired skin integrity
   —High risk for infection
   —High risk for injury
   —High risk for poisoning
   —High risk for trauma
   Higher level:
   —Altered thought processes
   —Anxiety
   —Decisional conflict (specify)
   —Fear
   —Ineffective denial
   —Ineffective family coping: disabling
   —Ineffective family coping: compromised
   —Ineffective individual coping
   —Ineffective management of therapeutic regimen (individual)
   —Knowledge deficit (specify)
   —Noncompliance (specify)

—High risk for violence: self-directed or directed at other
—High risk for self-mutilation
—Post-trauma response
—Rape-trauma syndrome
—Rape-trauma syndrome: compound reaction
—Rape-trauma syndrome: silent reaction
—Relocation stress syndrome

10. **Love and Belonging Needs**
—Altered family processes
—Altered parenting
—High risk for altered parenting
—Anticipatory grieving
—Caregiver role strain
—High risk for caregiver role strain
—Dysfunctional grieving
—Impaired social interaction
—Impaired verbal communication
—Parental role conflict
—Social isolation

11. **Spiritual Needs**
—Spiritual distress (distress of the human spirit)

12. **Self-Esteem Needs**
—Altered role performance
—Bathing/hygiene/self-care deficit
—Body image disturbance
—Chronic low self-esteem
—Defensive coping
—Dressing/grooming self-care deficit
—Hopelessness
—Personal identity disturbance
—Powerlessness
—Self-esteem disturbance
—Situational low self-esteem

13. **Self-Actualization Needs**
—Altered growth and development
—Family coping: potential for growth
—Health-seeking behaviors (specify)
—Impaired adjustment

Adapted from: *NANDA Nursing Diagnoses: Definitions and Classification 1992–1993.* Philadelphia, North American Nursing Diagnosis Association, 1992, with permission.

Mrs. Jones has complained of feeling frequent needs to void even at intervals of shorter duration than a movie. Thus, the nursing diagnosis of reflex incontinence is inaccurate. For the nursing diagnosis of stress incontinence, the major defining characteristic is reported dribbling of urine with increased abdominal pressure. A minor characteristic is urinary frequency more often

TABLE 3-2   APPROVED NANDA NURSING DIAGNOSTIC CATEGORIES. LISTED BY
HUMAN RESPONSE PATTERN.*

Pattern 1: Exchanging
   Altered nutrition: More than body requirements
   Altered nutrition: Less than body requirements
   Altered nutrition: Potential for more than body requirements
   High risk for infection
   High risk for altered body temperature
   Hypothermia
   Hyperthermia
   Ineffective thermoregulation
   Dysreflexia
   Constipation
   Perceived constipation
   Colonic constipation
   Diarrhea
   Bowel incontinence
   Altered urinary elimination
   Stress incontinence
   Reflex incontinence
   Urge incontinence
   Functional incontinence
   Total incontinence
   Urinary retention
   Altered tissue perfusion (specify type—renal, cerebral cardiopulmonary,
      gastrointestinal, peripheral)
   Fluid volume excess
   Fluid volume deficit
   High risk for fluid volume deficit
   Decreased cardiac output
   Impaired gas exchange
   Ineffective airway clearance
   Ineffective breathing pattern
   Inability to sustain spontaneous ventilation
   Dysfunctional ventilatory weaning response (DVWR)
   High risk for injury
   High risk for suffocation
   High risk for poisoning
   High risk for trauma
   High risk for aspiration
   High risk for disuse syndrome
   Altered protection
   Impaired tissue integrity
   Altered oral mucous membrane
   Skin integrity

Imparied high risk for imparied skin integrity
Pattern 2: Communicating
Impaired verbal communication
Pattern 3: Relating
Impaired social interaction
Social isolation
Altered role performance
Altered parenting
High risk for altered parenting
Sexual dysfunction
Altered family processes
Caregiver role strain
High risk for caregiver role strain
Parental role conflict
Altered sexuality patterns
Pattern 4: Valuing
Spiritual distress (distress of the human spirit)
Pattern 5: Choosing
Ineffective individual coping
Impaired adjustment
Defensive coping
Ineffective denial
Ineffective family coping: disabling
Ineffective family coping: compromised
Family coping: potential for growth
Ineffective management of therapeutic regimen
    (individuals)
Noncompliance (specify)
Decisional conflict (specify)
Health-seeking behaviors (specify)
Pattern 6: Moving
Impaired physical mobility
High risk for peripheral neurovascular dysfunction
Activity intolerance
Fatigue
High risk for activity intolerance
Sleep pattern disturbance
Diversional activity deficit
Impaired home maintenance management
Altered health maintenance
Feeding self-care deficit
Impaired swallowing
Ineffective breastfeeding
Interrupted breastfeeding
Effective breastfeeding
Ineffective infant feeding pattern

Bathing/hygiene self care deficit
Dressing/grooming self care deficit
Toileting self care deficit
Altered growth and development
Relocation stress syndrome
Pattern 7: Perceiving
Altered self-concept
Body image disturbance
Self-esteem disturbance
Chronic low self-esteem
Situational low self-esteem
Personal identity disturbance
Sensory/perceptual alterations (specify) (visual, auditory, kinesthetic,
    gustatory, tactile, olfactory)
Unilateral neglect
Hopelessness
Powerlessness
Pattern 8: Knowing
Knowledge deficit (specify)
Altered thought processes
Pattern 9: Feeling
Pain
Chronic pain
Dysfunctional grieving
Anticipatory grieving
High risk for violence: self directed or directed at others
High risk for self mutilation
Post-trauma response
Rape-trauma syndrome
Rape-trauma syndrome: compound reaction
Rape-trauma syndrome: silent reaction
Anxiety
Fear

Source: *NANDA Nursing Diagnoses: Definitions and Classification 1992–1993.* Philadelphia, North American Nursing Diagnosis Association, 1992, with permission.

than every two hours. Both of these characteristics match the symptoms reported by Mrs. Jones, and the nurse may reliably make the nursing diagnosis of stress incontinence.

FORMULATING THE NURSING DIAGNOSIS

The final activity in the process of diagnosing is the formulation of the nursing diagnosis.

The definition of a nursing diagnosis states that the problems the nurse chooses to address are within the scope of the legal practice of nursing, since this assumption underlies all professional activity. The privileges granted by licensure vary from state to state, country to country. Nurses with advanced degrees may be licensed to perform additional nursing care. However, all professional nurses share the responsibility of making nursing diagnoses within their practice.

A nursing diagnosis is not the same as a medical diagnosis though it may involve the medical diagnosis or treatment as a cause. For example, the nursing diagnosis of *pain* is clearly related to the medical diagnosis in many cases: pain may be caused by a surgical incision, by cancer which has metastasized to the bones, by stones in the gallbladder. However, since nurses cannot treat the medical diagnosis, the direction for nursing diagnosis must then come from the problem part of the statement. Table 3-3 clarifies nursing diagnoses. A medical diagnosis frequently suggests nursing diagnoses. The experienced nurse who has cared for several clients with the same medical diagnosis will be able to predict some frequently occurring nursing diagnoses for a given medical condition. The nurse is then looking for data to validate the prediction. This experience contributes to skill in making nursing diagnoses. Table 3-4 gives examples of nursing diagnoses which are suggested by medical diagnoses.

The nurse begins the process of writing nursing diagnoses by reviewing the problem focus area identified in the previous step. Does the focus area represent a problem? By definition, a diagnosis must be a problem for the client. If it is not a problem, no diagnosis need be made. Consider the bowel function status of a client restricted to bed rest. If the client has a soft, formed stool without exertion every two or three days, elimination is not a problem and no nursing diagnosis need be made. However, the nurse also considers who defines the problem. If the client considers it abnormal not to have a bowel movement daily and continues to express anxiety related to this, a problem does exist as defined by the client. The nurse understands that physiologically no problem exists, but that the client could benefit from teaching regarding normal body function. Nursing care may then focus on teaching as an intervention tool to reduce anxiety. Nursing diagnoses may also identify growth areas for the client. Many nurses in industrial health or occupational health nursing report that the clients they see are requesting ways to improve their health status. While this does not constitute a problem, it is a focus area for nursing intervention. Tripp and Stachowiak (1989) have proposed a nursing diagnosis that would label this as "health-seeking behavior." This nursing diagnosis does clearly identify an area of nursing intervention that is not a problem in the negative sense.

Types of Nursing Diagnoses

ACTUAL NURSING DIAGNOSES.   As defined here, the problem expressed in the nursing diagnosis may be either actual or high risk. An *actual nursing diagnosis*

TABLE 3-3   A NURSING DIAGNOSIS

Is	Is Not
A statement of a client problem	A medical diagnosis
Actual, high risk, or possible	A nursing action
Within the scope of nursing practice	A physician order
Directive of nursing intervention	A therapeutic treatment

refers to a problem existing at the present moment; existing in reality (Carroll-Johnson, 1991). A client on a general diet with a good appetite has not had a bowel movement for four days, complains of low abdominal pain, and is unable to pass stool. The client is constipated and requires nursing assistance. This situation requires that an actual nursing diagnosis be made.

HIGH-RISK NURSING DIAGNOSES.   A *high-risk nursing diagnosis* is a clinical judgment that an individual, family, or community is more vulnerable to develop the problem than others in the same or similar situation. The nurse has identified factors in either the admission data base or in ongoing assessments that indicate risk factors for the development of a problem. If a client is on bed rest following total hip replacement, complains of pain on movement, and is poorly nourished, the client is at high risk for skin breakdown (decubitus ulcers). Understanding the physiological effect of prolonged bed rest, the nurse will implement interventions to prevent skin breakdown. In this example, the problem is a high-risk one that requires preventive nursing action. The high-risk nursing diagnosis is made based on the nurse's learning and past experience in similar situations and on an understanding of pathophysiology. The problem would predictably occur without nursing intervention.

TABLE 3-4   MEDICAL DIAGNOSES THAT SUGGEST NURSING DIAGNOSES

Medical Diagnosis	Nursing Diagnosis
Myocardial infarction	Fear related to possible recurrence and uncertain outcome
Chronic ulcerative colitis	Diarrhea related to CUC as manifested by 10–12 loose, watery, foul smelling stools per day
Chronic ulcerative colitis	Alteration in nutrition: less than body requirements related to altered G.I. absorption secondary to CUC
Cancer of the breast	High risk for body image disturbance if mastectomy is required
Cerebral vascular accident	Self-care deficit: dressing and grooming related to right-sided flaccidity

POSSIBLE NURSING DIAGNOSES.   In still other situations the nurse may decide to formulate a tentative or *possible nursing diagnosis*. This may be compared to the physician who lists several "rule out" medical diagnoses in a client's admission assessment. The physician may then order diagnostic tests to gather more data to make a decision. So it is with a possible nursing diagnosis. By considering a possible nursing diagnosis, the nurse assures continued collection of relevant data. With an increased data base, the nurse may be able to firmly establish the possible nursing diagnosis as valid or to eliminate it as invalid for a particular client. For example:

> While caring for a postpartum client who has delivered a baby born with a cleft lip a few hours before, the nurse anticipates a possible nursing diagnosis of dysfunctional grieving. The nurse hypothesizes that the client might be feeling guilty, be crying, be angry and sad. The nurse enters the client's room and after introducing herself, observes the new mother holding the infant and visually and tactilely exploring the infant's body. The mother speaks gently and warmly to the infant. The nurse comments to the client, "How are you doing with your daughter?" The client replies, "Well, for a brief moment I was upset with the cleft, but I think my doctor was more upset than I was! You see, I am a nurse also. I work with a plastic surgeon, and I have seen literally hundreds of these conditions. This is nothing! In a couple of months this will be repaired and it will be impossible to see that anything was wrong. I really trust the surgeon I work for. I can handle this. What if it had been something serious?" At this point the nurse can rule out the possible nursing diagnosis based on the data: maternal bonding, verbal statements of the mother, tactile exploration of the baby's body, nonverbal language of the mother.

COLLABORATIVE PROBLEMS

Some nurses also distinguish between nursing diagnoses that the nurse treats independently and those which the nurse treats collaboratively (jointly shared) with the physician. Nursing and medicine are complementary to each other. Physicians rely on nurses to understand and assess for physiological complications related to clients' medical treatments such as postsurgical phlebitis. The nurse and the physician discuss the problem and the physician will order new treatments, medications, or intensive monitoring. The nurse carries out these medical orders and continues assessment that is reported to the physician. These types of problems are collaborative. The nurse in this situation is not licensed to prescribe the primary treatment needed to resolve the problem. Much of the assessment and treatment of the problem is directed by the physician even though the nurse may carry it out and adapt it to the particular client situation. This is interdependent nursing practice. A large part of nursing care involves this kind of collaborative assessment and intervention. In contrast, the independent role of the nurse deals with how the client responds to actual or high-risk health problems. The nurse not only monitors the client for these problems but is licensed to diagnose, prescribe, and carry out treatment for these problems. This text considers both independent and interdependent components of nursing practice.

Many nursing diagnoses have both an independent aspect and a collaborative component. For example, there are many measures the nurse may independently use to assist the client in pain (massage, guided imagery, relaxation techniques), although it is usually a physician's prerogative to order a medication. (Some states permit nurse practitioners this practice privilege.) This is an example of a collaborative problem that incorporates independent nursing functions. Other collaborative problems are primarily within the realm of medicine, and the nurse monitors the client and reports to the physician for medical diagnoses and treatment. Fluid volume deficit is being discussed as such a collaborative problem. Even though this is a NANDA-approved nursing diagnosis, much of the treatment is determined by the physician and implemented by the nurse. The physician orders the IV and electrolyte replacement, diet therapy, and activity levels, but the nurse is responsible for the implementation. Much of the work of staff nurses in hospitals involves a collaborative role not only with physicians but with professionals in many other disciplines. Nurses share a collaborative role with therapeutic dieticians to resolve the nutritional problems of clients. Psychiatric nurses identify collaborative problems with dance therapists, music therapists, and occupational therapists. The collaborative role is not unique to the disciplines of nursing and medicine.

In addition to deciding if the focus area represents a problem for the client, the nurse considers a second criterion: Does the problem require nursing intervention to be resolved, lessened, or accommodated? The nurse may identify problems that are clearly within the realm of another health professional. In such a case, the nurse communicates the data to that professional and does not make a diagnosis.

Writing Nursing Diagnoses

ACTUAL NURSING DIAGNOSES.   The following formula will result in a clear, concise statement of an *actual (or present) nursing diagnosis*:

$$\text{Actual Nursing Diagnosis} = \text{Client Problem} + \text{Cause if Known}$$

When writing the diagnosis, the nurse usually replaces the plus symbol with the words "related to," which are abbreviated "r/t." The following are examples of nursing diagnoses in this format:

Actual Nursing Diagnoses		
Problem	*+*	*Cause*
1. Impaired skin integrity	r/t	physical immobilization
2. Parental role conflict	r/t	divorce
3. Impaired verbal communication	r/t	inability to speak dominant language

This is a very clear and concise way of writing nursing diagnoses. This is the way nursing diagnoses will usually be written in the hospital. The nurse may not always know the cause of the problem, and in such a case may simply write "cause unknown."

PES Format. There is another format used for writing actual nursing diagnoses, one which may be especially helpful for beginning nursing students. Using this approach, which is referred to as PES (Gordon, 1982), the formula for a nursing diagnosis would look like this:

PES APPROACH

$$\text{Nursing Diagnosis} = \frac{P + E + S}{\text{Problem} + \text{Etiology} + \text{Signs \& Symptoms}}$$

Using this formula the nurse first selects the approved NANDA nursing diagnosis and then relates it to the cause, which is the same as the etiology. The signs and symptoms describe the problem, not the etiology. NANDA (1989) suggests signs and symptoms associated with specific nursing diagnoses under the headings: defining characteristics. The characteristics are grouped according to frequency of occurrence. *Critical defining characteristics* must be present for the diagnosis to be made. *Major defining characteristics* appear to be present in all clients experiencing the problem. *Minor defining characteristics* appear to be present in many clients experiencing the problem (NANDA, 1989, p. 560). Demonstrating the presence of the critical and major defining characteristics greatly increases the accuracy of the nursing diagnosis. This may be very helpful to the beginning student, although practicing professional nurses do not often use this longer format. The following would be examples of the same actual nursing diagnoses as above written in the PES format:

1. Impaired skin integrity related to physical immobilization as manifested by disruption of the skin surface over the elbows and coccyx.

2. Parental role conflict related to divorce as manifested by statements of unsatisfactory child care during working hours.
3. Impaired verbal communication related to cultural differences as manifested by inability to speak English.

HIGH-RISK NURSING DIAGNOSES.   For a *high-risk nursing diagnosis* the nurse uses the following format:

$$\begin{matrix} \text{High-Risk} \\ \text{Nursing Diagnosis} \end{matrix} = \text{Problem} + \text{Risk Factors}$$

When making a high-risk nursing diagnosis the nurse is unable to list the signs and symptoms because the problem has not yet developed; and in fact, the nurse will attempt to intervene so the problem does not occur. Here the nurse lists the risk factors that have been identified from the assessment that indicate the problem is very likely to occur. The following are examples of high-risk nursing diagnoses:

High-Risk Nursing Diagnoses		
Problem	+	*Risk Factor*
1. Skin breakdown: high-risk	r/t	physical immobilization in total body cast
2. Fluid volume deficit: high-risk	r/t	diarrhea, age 3 yrs, low oral intake, elevated temperature
3. Injury: high-risk	r/t	disorientation and decreased vision after (cataract) surgery

POSSIBLE NURSING DIAGNOSES.   The nurse may write a *possible nursing diagnosis* as an incomplete problem statement since the validity of the problem is uncertain but considered a possibility, based on the way many clients respond to similar situations or conditions. Because the purpose of this diagnosis is to assure continued data collection, it is not possible at this stage to identify either signs or symptoms or risk factors. The nurse would merely state:

Possible sensory-perceptual alteration
Possible nutritional deficit
Possible fluid volume deficit

Each of these diagnoses requires that the nurse continue to collect sufficient data to make a decision regarding the existence of a nursing problem in this area.

The nurse is now ready to begin writing nursing diagnoses. The following steps summarize the process:

1. Review the assessment data.
2. Identify the problem focus area.
3. Consult NANDA listing of nursing diagnoses to aid in stating the problem. Match the client's signs and symptoms with the defining characteristics of diagnoses in the problem focus area. Select the diagnosis with the best match.
4. State the cause if known.
5. State the signs, symptoms, risk factors if appropriate.

Occasionally the student will describe a problem that is not included in the NANDA listing. This may reflect an accurate problem. Nursing is an evolving science and the listing of nursing diagnoses is in the process of development. When this happens the nurse states the problem as clearly and as concisely as possible in a way that communicates the problem to those involved in the care of the client. The nurse may wish to inform NANDA of this finding and follow the procedure for submitting a new diagnosis for approval and clinical testing.

Validating Nursing Diagnoses

When the nurse has completed writing the nursing diagnoses, the ANA *Standards of Clinical Nursing Practice* require that they are validated with the client, and with significant others and health care providers, when possible. This need not be a formal or lengthy session, but the nurse must assure that it occurs. For example, the nurse might bring the care plan to the client and indicate, "Mrs. Jones, I have identified some health care problems that I will be using to plan nursing care during your hospitalization. Could you please help me by telling me if you agree with what I have identified, or if I have perhaps missed some that are important to you?" This offers clients the opportunity to participate in and make decisions about their care.

NURSING DIAGNOSIS: THE NEXT GENERATION

The nurse who is practicing in a setting where case management is practiced still uses and is accountable for the diagnosis step of the nursing process. This nurse has the professional responsibility to conduct and document a nursing assessment. The nurse then may use a form such as a CareMap® (Zander, 1991) that identifies nursing diagnoses related to a particular medical diagnosis and DRG. The nursing diagnoses identified in the CareMap® have been established by expert nurses and have been found to be valid for the vast majority of clients with a particular medical diagnosis.

The staff nurse uses the documented nursing assessment to validate that the nursing diagnoses of the CareMap® are appropriate to this particular client. It may be necessary to add or delete nursing diagnoses to make the CareMap® appropriate for an individual client. One way of doing this might be to add the etiologies of the particular client to the nursing diagnoses. See Table 3-5 for a CareMap® example. The nursing diagnoses, numbered 1 through 7, are listed under the "Problem" heading on the upper left side of the CareMap.®

SUMMARY

The process of diagnosing consists of three activities: data analysis, problem identification, and the formulation of nursing diagnoses. During data analysis the nurse makes decisions based on the data regarding the health status of the client. Next the nurse identifies problem focus areas and finally states a nursing diagnosis. The nursing diagnosis includes the client problem and cause or etiology if known. The statement may also include signs and symptoms *if* the student is using the PES format. If the client is at high risk for developing a certain problem, the nurse makes a high-risk nursing diagnosis and includes the identification of risk factors that determined the diagnosis.

PRACTICE EXERCISE

Pick out the correctly written nursing diagnoses. Identify what is wrong with the incorrectly written nursing diagnoses. (Either the abbreviated formula or the PES formula is acceptable.) The correct answers follow the exercise.

1. Alteration in nutrition: less than body requirements related to nausea following chemotherapy.
2. Range of motion exercises (ROM) following a cerebral vascular accident (CVA).
3. Cancer of the breast with metastasis to the axillary lymph nodes.
4. Refusing wound irrigation related to pain of procedure.
5. Body image disturbance related to amputation of right foot.
6. Potential for sexual dysfunction in relating to husband and friends related to mastectomy.
7. Intermittent positive pressure breathing (IPPB) exercises q.i.d. to increase lung expansion
8. Pain and fear related to surgical procedure.
9. Severe itching related to a fungal infection.

TABLE 3-5 CAREMAP®: CONGESTIVE HEART FAILURE

	Day 1	Day 1	Day 2	Day 3	Day 4	Day 5	Day 6
			Benchmark Quality Criteria				
Location	ER 1–4 hours	Floor Telemetry or CCU 6–24 hours	Floor	Floor	Floor	Floor	Floor
Problem							
1) Alteration in gas exchange/ profusion and fluid balance due to decreased cardiac output, excess fluid volume	Reduced pain from admission or pain free Uses pain scale O_2 sat. improved over admission baseline on O_2 therapy	Respirations equal to or less than on admission	O_2 sat = 90 Resp 20–22 Vital signs stable Crackles at lung bases Mild shortness of breath with activity	Does not require O_2 Vital signs stable Crackles at base Respirations 20–22 Mild shortness of breath with activity	Does not require O_2 (O_2 sat. on room air 90%) Vital signs stable Crackles at base Respirations 20–22 Completes activities with no increase in respirations No edema	Can lie in bed at baseline position Chest X-ray clear or at baseline	No dyspnea
2) Potential for shock	No signs/ symptoms of shock	No signs/ symptoms of shock	No signs/ symptoms of shock	No signs/ symptoms of shock Normal lab values	No signs/ symptoms of shock	No signs/ symptoms of shock	No signs/ symptoms of shock
3) Potential for consequences of immobility and decreased	No redness at pressure points No falls	No redness at pressure points No falls	Tolerates chair, washing, eating, and toileting	Has bowel movement Up in room and bathroom with	Up ad lib for short periods	Activity increased to level used at home without	Activity increased to level used at home without

52

activity: skin breakdown. DVT				assist		shortness of breath	shortness of breath
4) Alteration in nutritional intake due to nausea and vomiting, labored		No c/o nausea No vomiting Taking liquids as offered	Eating solids Takes in 50% each meal	Taking 50% each meal	Taking 50% each meal Weight 2 lbs from patient's normal baseline	Taking 75% each meal	Taking 75% each meal
5) Potential for arrhythmias due to decreased cardiac output: decreased irritable foci, valve problems, decreased gas exchange	No evidence of life-threatening dysrhythmias	Normal sinus rhythm with benign ectopy	K(WNL) Benign or no arrhythmias	Digoxin level WNL Benign or no arrhythmias	Digoxin level WNL Benign or no arrhythmias	Digoxin level WNL Benign or no arrhythmias	Digoxin level WNL Benign or no arrhythmias
6) Patient/family response to future treatment & hospitalization	Patient/family expressing concerns Following directions of staff	Patient/family expressing concerns Following directions of staff	Patient/family expressing concerns Following directions of staff	States reasons for and cooperates with rest periods Patient begins to assess own knowledge and ability to care for CHF at home	Patient decides whether he/she wants discussion with physician about advanced directives	States plan for 1–2 days post-discharge as to meds., diet, activity, follow-up appointments Expresses reaction to having CHF	Repeats plans States signs and symptoms to notify physician/ER Signs discharge consent

TABLE 3-5 CAREMAP®: CONGESTIVE HEART FAILURE (Continued)

	Day 1	Day 1	Day 2	Day 3	Day 4	Day 5	Day 6
	ER 1–4 hours	Floor Telemetry or CCU 6–24 hours		*Benchmark Quality Criteria*			
Location			*Floor*	*Floor*	*Floor*	*Floor*	*Floor*
Problem							
7) Individual problem:							
Staff Tasks							
Assessments/ Consults	Vital signs q 15 min; Nursing assessments focus on lung sounds, edema, color, skin integrity, jugular vein distention; Cardiac monitor; Arterial line if needed; Swan Ganz; Intake & output	Vital signs q 15 min–1 hr; Repeat nursing assessments; Cardiac monitor; Arterial line; Swan Ganz; Daily weight; Intake & output	Vital signs q 4 hrs; Repeat nursing assessments; D/C cardiac monitor 24 hr; D/C arterial and Swan Ganz; Daily weight; Intake & output	Vital signs q 6 hrs; Repeat nursing assessments; Daily weight; Intake & output	Vital signs q 6 hrs; Repeat nursing assessments; Daily weight; Intake & output; Nutrition consult	Vital signs q 6 hrs; Repeat nursing assessments; Daily weight; Intake & output	Vital signs q 6 hrs; Repeat nursing assessments; Daily weight; Intake & output
Specimens/Tests	Consider TSH studies; Chest X-ray; EKG; CPK q 8 hr × 3; ABG if pulse Ox: (range)	B/G	Evaluate for ECHO; Lytes, BUN, Creatinine			Chest X-ray; Lytes, BUN, Creatinine	

	Lytes, Na, K, Cl, CO$_2$ Glucose, BUN, Creatinine Digoxin: (range)						
Treatments	O$_2$ or intubate IV or Heparin lock	O$_2$ IV or Heparin lock	IV or Heparin lock	DC pulse Ox if stable D/C IV or Heparin lock			
Medications	Evaluate for Digoxin Nitrodrip or paste Diuretics IV	Evaluate for Digoxin Nitrodrip or paste	D/C Nitrodrip or paste Diuretics IV or PO	Change to PODigoxin PO diuretics	PO diuretics K supplement Stool softeners	PO diuretics K supplement Stool softeners	PO diuretics K supplement Stool softeners
	Evaluate for antiemetics Evaluate for antiarrhythmics	Diuretics IV Evaluate for pre-load/after-load reducers K supplements Stool softeners	K supplements Stool softeners Evaluate for nicotine patch	K supplements Stool softeners Nicotine patch if consent	Nicotine patch if consent	Nicotine patch if consent	Nicotine patch if consent
Nutrition	None	Clear liquids	Cardiac, low-salt diet	Cardiac, low-salt diet	Cardiac, low-salt diet	Cardiac, low-salt diet	Cardiac, low-salt diet
Safety/Activity	Commode Bedrest with head elevated Reposition patient q 2 hrs Bedrails up Call light available	Commode Bedrest with head elevated Dangle Reposition patient q 2 hrs Enforce rest periods Bedrails up Call light available	Commode Enforce rest periods Chair with assist ½ hr with feet elevated Bedrails up Call light available	Bathroom privileges Chair × 3 Bedrails up Call light available	Ambulate in hall × 2 Up ad lib between rest periods Bedrails up Call light available	Encourage ADLs that approximate activities at home Bedrails up Call light available	Encourage ADLs that approximate activities at home Bedrails up Call light available

TABLE 3-5   CAREMAP®: CONGESTIVE HEART FAILURE (*Continued*)

	Day 1	Day 1	Day 2	Day 3	Day 4	Day 5	Day 6
				Benchmark Quality Criteria			
Location	ER 1–4 hours	Floor Telemetry or CCU 6–24 hours	Floor	Floor	Floor	Floor	Floor
Staff Tasks							
Teaching	Explain procedures Teach chest pain scale and importance of reporting	Explain course, need for energy conservation Orient to unit and routine	Clarify CHF Dx and future teaching needs Orient to unit and routine Schedule rest periods Begin medication teaching	Importance of weighing self every day Provide smoking cessation information Review energy conservation schedule	Cardiac rehab level as indicated by consult Provide smoking cessation support Dietary teaching	Review CHF education material with patient	Reinforce CHF teaching
Transfer/Discharge Coordination	Assess home situation: notify significant other If no arrhythmias or chest pain, transfer to floor Otherwise transfer to ICU	Screen for discharge needs Transfer to floor	Consider Home Health Care referral		Evaluate needs for diet and anti-smoking classes Physician offers discussion opportunities for advanced directives	Appointment and arrangement for follow-up care with Home Health Care nurses Contact VNA	Reinforce follow-up appointments

Reproduced by permission. CareMap® is a registered trademark and intellectual property of the Center for Case Management, South Natick, MA.

10. Activity intolerance related to shortness of breath on activity.
11. Impaired physical mobility associated with right sided paralysis.
12. Ineffective breathing pattern etiology unknown, as evidenced by shortness of breath, tachypnea, pursed lip breathing.
13. Disorientation to time and place related to confused state.
14. Impaired verbal communication related to inability to speak dominant English language.
15. Fear related to uncertain outcome of surgery as manifested by urinary frequency, irritability, rapid pulse, "It's all I can think about—I'm sure it's cancer."
16. Ambulate progressively with tripod cane.
17. High risk for infection related to second degree burns on right hand.
18. Client is upset and worried about the cost of hospitalization.
19. Impaired skin integrity related to prolonged bed rest as manifested by skin breakdown over both elbows and coccyx.
20. Thrombophlebitis related to prolonged bed rest as manifested by a positive Homan's sign.

ANSWERS TO EXERCISE ON NURSING DIAGNOSIS

1. Correct.   Problem= less than body requirements for nutritional needs
              Cause   = nausea following chemotherapy
   In this case nursing care will focus on methods to relieve the nausea.
2. Incorrect.
   Range of motion exercises are a nursing intervention.
3. Incorrect.
   Cancer of the breast is a medical diagnosis, one which the nurse is not licensed to treat. The experienced nurse might anticipate possible nursing diagnoses having to do with pain, body image, fear, or anxiety.
4. Incorrect.
   This is a nursing problem. The real nursing diagnosis may be something like: Pain associated with irrigation procedure. There would be many things the nurse could do to deal with the pain and make the procedure more acceptable to the client.
5. Correct.   Problem= body image disturbance
              Cause   = amputation of the right foot
6. Correct.   Problem= potential for sexual dysfunction
              Cause   = related to mastectomy
7. Incorrect. This is a medical treatment.
8. Incorrect. These are two separate problems that will each require different nursing care.
9. Correct.   Problem= severe itching
              Cause   = fungal infection

While this diagnosis is not listed in a NANDA format it does clearly convey the client problem. However, the nurse does need additional information regarding the location of the infection. In this case the PES format would be helpful. The signs and symptoms might include: client complaints, scratch marks and rash on right leg, restlessness.

10. Incorrect. SOB is not a cause but a sign/symptom. Need etiology if known in diagnostic statement.

11. Correct.

12. Correct.   P= ineffective breathing pattern
    E= unknown
    S= shortness of breath, tachypnea, pursed-lip breathing

13. Incorrect. Problem and cause are the same.

14. Correct.   Problem= impaired verbal communication
    Cause   = inability to speak dominant English language

15. Correct.   P= anxiety
    E= uncertain outcome of surgery
    S= urinary frequency, irritability, rapid pulse, "It's all I can think about—I'm sure it's cancer."

16. Incorrect. This is a physician's order.

17. Correct.   Problem= high risk for infection
    Cause   = related to second degree burns on right hand

18. Incorrect. This is a judgment. It may indicate that there is a problem, but additional data are needed. This may be a problem that the nurse will refer to a social worker who has additional resources to assist this client.

19. Correct.   P= impaired skin integrity
    E= related to prolonged bed rest
    S= skin breakdown over coccyx and both elbows

20. Incorrect. This is a medical diagnosis, but it would suggest possible nursing diagnoses related to physical safety and pain. These would need further client data for confirmation.

CASE STUDY: NURSING DIAGNOSES

The case study of Mrs. Witten is continued from Chapter 2 to identify nursing diagnoses. The NANDA-approved diagnostic categories are used. Two different formats are used for stating the diagnosis of an actual problem. The first format uses the three parts: problem identification, etiology, and signs and symptoms of the problem (PES format). The second format uses two parts: problem identification and etiology. The signs and symptoms are listed under the category of "supporting data."

Mrs. Witten: Nursing Diagnoses

Example 1.

a. Pain related to possible gallbladder disease as evidenced by verbal report of RUQ pain, restlessness, elevated pulse and respirations.

b. Pain related to possible gallbladder disease.

   supporting data: c/o acute pain in RUQ; pulse 95, respirations 28, restless and clenching hands, gritting teeth, admitting medical diagnosis is to rule out cholecystitis

Example 2.

a. Fear related to illness and possible surgery/laparoscopic cholecystectomy as evidenced by report of being "scared," elevated pulse and respirations, crying, and muscle tension.

b. Fear related to illness and possible surgery/laparoscopic cholecystectomy.

   supporting data: reports feeling "scared"; states never been hospitalized; tears in eyes; pulse 96; diaphoretic (sweating); respirations 28; trembling hands

Example 3.

a. Altered health maintenance related to lack of knowledge and skill in breast self-exam (BSE) as evidenced by statement of not doing BSE because it was never learned.

b. Altered health maintenance related to lack of knowledge and skill in BSE.

   supporting data: reports she does not do BSE; states "never learned"

CHAPTER 4

Planning

STANDARD III. OUTCOME IDENTIFICATION

The Nurse Identifies Expected Outcomes Individualized to the Client.

STANDARD IV. PLANNING

The Nurse Develops a Plan of Care That Prescribes Interventions to Attain Expected Outcomes.

Standards of Care in *Standards of Clinical Nursing Practice*, American Nurses Association, 1991. Used by permission.

Now that the nurse has collected data about a client, analyzed that data, and formulated some nursing diagnoses, the planning phase of the nursing process begins. In the planning phase, the nurse develops a plan to assist the client to an optimum or improved level of functioning in the problem areas identified in the nursing diagnoses. The nurse analyzes the strengths and weaknesses of the client, the client's family, the nursing personnel, the health care facility, and the available resources (including other health care professionals). The nurse also examines personal strengths, beliefs, and values that might affect the care planning phase. A nurse who is unable or unwilling to work with a client in a particular problem area may need to seek help from another more experienced staff nurse, clinical instructor, or other resource.

A plan is developed to make nursing care both individualized for the client and realistic for the hospital or home care setting. The skills of problem solving and decision making are applied to a particular client's identified problems. The resulting plan of nursing care is designed to help clients and their families:

—maintain their current level of health and functioning if they are identified at risk for developing problems

—avoid injury or disease
—regain a previous level of health and functioning
—reach an improved level of health and functioning
—adjust to reduced level of health and functioning when improvement is not possible
—adjust to a progressively decreasing level of functioning when terminally ill

The following areas for nursing care are identified by the American Nurses Association in their 1991 *Standards of Clinical Nursing Practice* as:

- Disease or injury prevention
- Health promotion
- Health restoration
- Health maintenance

ACTIVITIES IN THE PLANNING PHASE

There are three steps in the planning phase: setting priorities among the nursing diagnoses when a client has several problems, establishing outcomes with a client, and planning specific nursing interventions to help a client achieve the outcomes.

$$\text{Planning} = \frac{\text{Setting}}{\text{Priorities}} + \frac{\text{Establishing}}{\text{Outcomes}} + \frac{\text{Planning}}{\text{Nursing}} \\ \text{Interventions}$$

SETTING PRIORITIES

During the process of priority setting, the nurse and the client, whenever possible, mutually determine which problems identified during the assessment phase are in need of immediate attention and which problems might be dealt with at a later time. Consider assigning identified client problems a high, middle, or low priority. The higher priority problems deserve the most immediate nursing attention for a plan and treatment. Setting priorities serves the purpose of ordering the delivery of nursing care so that more important or life threatening problems are treated before less critical problems. Priority setting does not mean that one problem must be totally resolved before another problem is considered. Problems can frequently be approached simultaneously. At times, decreasing the severity of one problem works to eliminate the others, as when eliminating severe pain corrects an ineffective breathing pattern.

Guidelines for Setting Priorities

1. Maslow's hierarchy of basic needs can guide the selection of high-priority problems. Survival needs that are significantly unmet pose the greatest threat to life and functioning and thus deserve a high-priority rating. Using Maslow's theory to guide the delivery of nursing care, the nurse would:
   —Relieve a client's pain (physiological need) before encouraging morning hygiene (self-esteem)
   —Encourage a new mother to express her disappointment about having a C-section when she had planned on totally natural childbirth (self-esteem) before teaching her infant care skills (self-actualization)
   —Stabilize bleeding and ensure adequate oxygenation in an emergency room accident victim before assessing elimination status (both of these are basic physiological needs, but oxygenation is usually the highest priority need; bleeding is considered a threat to tissue oxygenation)
   —Consider how difficult it is for you to read and absorb the material in this book (self-actualization need) if you have had too little sleep (physiological need)

   Basic survival needs will usually take priority over higher level needs if the survival needs are not being satisfied. This is the case when a client is in obvious physical distress owing to the unmet need. If the survival needs are being partially met and actual physical distress is tolerable, a higher level need may take priority, or at least have the same priority as a lower level need. For example, an auto accident victim can be in considerable distress with multiple physical needs unmet, yet the priority need may be to ascertain the whereabouts and injuries of the other family members in the car when it crashed. This unmet higher level need can have a negative effect on satisfaction of this client's physical needs if it is not given appropriate attention.

2. Focus on the problems the client feels are most important if this priority does not interfere with medical treatment. A client's need for undisturbed rest cannot take precedence over a medically ordered treatment for observation of blood pressure and pulse every hour following a car accident.

   If there are no nursing contraindications, offer clients the opportunity to set their own priorities. However, do not offer clients the opportunity to make choices they really do not have, or are not qualified to make. After surgery, the client and family may identify the need for rest and pain management as priority concerns, while the nurse is equally concerned about maintaining a clear airway and improving gas exchange based on an assessment of diminished breath sounds and moist gurgling heard in the lungs. The challenge for the nurse is to help all involved understand and agree about which problems will be dealt with now, and which problems may have to wait until the client is more stable.

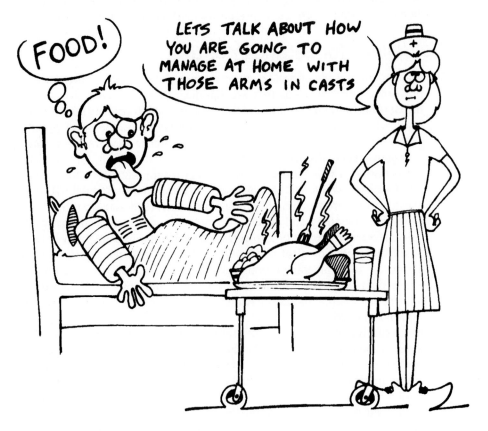

FIGURE 4-1. Priority setting.

Mutual priority setting with the client serves two purposes. First, this approach involves clients in planning their own care. Perhaps the nurse has overlooked a major problem that is consuming the client's time and energy or has assigned the problem a low priority. Unless this problem is considered first, the nurse may be able to achieve only limited success in other areas because the client is still worrying about the overlooked problem. Second, cooperation between the nurse and the client is enhanced when priority setting is done together. The nurse often acts as an interpreter by stating recognition of the client and family concerns, sharing nursing and medical concerns with the client/family, and guiding priority setting to promote safe physical care, attend to the client's concerns as soon as possible, and fit within the time and work constraints of the health care setting. The nurse also identifies client/family concerns to the physician, other nurses, and other health care professionals who may then reset their priorities based on a better understanding of the client's status.

3. Consider the client's culture, values, and beliefs when setting priorities.

Nurses are increasingly working with clients and families from cultures other than the dominant culture in which most nurses grew up and were educated. Clients may hold very different views of health and health care, and these beliefs cannot be ignored. Instead, they should be respected and considered in priority setting whenever possible.

4. Consider the effect of potential problems when setting priorities. For example:

—A new mother may ask to be left alone with her husband and newborn to get acquainted. The potential collaborative problem of a postpartum hemorrhage developing would require continuous observation after delivery, since this is potentially life threatening. Thus the client's request to be left alone cannot be safely met.

—A bedridden client may be started on a routine of frequent turning and positioning to prevent bed sores and contractures, even though the client may not see this as important. Prevention of the potential complications associated with prolonged bed rest is a high priority, since treating these problems after they develop is less effective, more costly, and usually more time-consuming than preventive measures.

Prevention of a high-risk problem, rather than treatment of the problem when it develops, is an outcome deserving continuous assessment and intervention.

5. Consider costs, resources available, personnel, and time needed to plan for and treat each of the client's identified problems. If resources, personnel, time, or financing is currently unavailable to deal with a particular problem, it may receive a low priority until some of these obstacles have been overcome. If a problem can be quickly resolved, it may receive a high priority for practical reasons.

6. Consider state laws, hospital policy statements, and outcome criteria established for the particular setting. For example, in many states it is the law that all children under the age of 4 years must be transported in an approved car seat. Hospital policy may state that newborns must be taken home by their parents in an appropriate car seat. This potential problem of injury to the newborn if not in a car seat during an automobile accident should be discussed early to give the family time to obtain a car seat before discharge.

ESTABLISHING OUTCOMES

The second step in the planning phase of the nursing process is to establish outcomes for each of the client's problems identified by the nursing diagnoses. An outcome is a "measurable, expected, client-focused goal" (ANA, 1991) to be achieved at some specified time in the future. For an *actual nursing diagnosis* where the problem currently exists, the outcome describes a future change in the client's health status or functioning showing a reduction or lessening of the problem. For a *high-risk nursing diagnosis*, which does not currently exist but has a high probability of occurring without preventive nursing interventions, the outcome is often to maintain the current problem-free status or level of functioning.

CLIENT OUTCOME
The desired result of nursing care; that which you hope to achieve with your client and which is designed to prevent, remedy, or lessen the problem identified in the nursing diagnosis.

Why Is an Outcome Statement Needed?

Outcomes are needed as part of the plan of care because they tell the nurse and the client where they are going. They should be part of the nurse's thinking whenever care is given. "Where am I going with this client today? Where do the client and I hope to be in relation to lessening or resolving a particular problem by the end of my shift?" The outcomes give guidance in the selection of nursing interventions. Outcomes are constant future targets to remind all caregivers and the client why certain activities or interventions are done. Outcomes give a standard against which to compare the client's hourly, daily, weekly, monthly, yearly, and lifelong efforts to maintain and improve health and functioning. Outcomes give a sense of where this particular client started from and where the individual and the nurse hope to end up. The assessment data provide the *baseline* for the client's current level of function in a problem area. For example, a newly diagnosed diabetic has lost 20 pounds, is dehydrated, and is inadequately nourished. The outcome might be for the individual to regain 15 lbs over the next two months, taking his prescribed amount of insulin each day. Progress toward this outcome over the weeks will be measured against the original baseline data and the optimal weight gain identified in the outcome statement. The outcomes nurses write will be the criteria used to evaluate the success of nursing interventions. An outcome helps to motivate both the nurse and the client to continue their efforts. When outcomes are achieved, it provides the client, the client's family, and the nurse and other caregivers with the reward of success, and success promotes further efforts to achieve additional, higher level outcomes.

The outcome for a student in nursing might be to graduate from school with a GPA of 3.0. Another student might set higher or lower outcome criteria depending on competing life responsibilities and personal abilities. The same is true in nursing practice. Without a clear, concise outcome statement, the nurse and the client do not know if and when the desired end has been achieved.

Components of an Outcome Statement

At least one outcome is written for each nursing diagnosis. Generally, several outcomes are written for each diagnosis, especially if there is a broad scope to the problem. Outcomes are written to include specific components that are identified in the box below.

$$\text{Outcome Statement} = \text{Client Behavior} + \text{Criteria of Performance} + \text{Conditions (if needed)} + \text{Time Frame}$$

CLIENT BEHAVIOR.   The client behavior the nurse selects for the outcome statement is an observable activity the client will demonstrate following a series of nursing interventions. The activity is observable in that it can be seen, heard, felt, or measured by the nurse. The activity chosen shows an improved level of functioning in the problem area identified in the nursing diagnosis. If the nursing diagnosis is a high-risk problem versus an actual current problem, the activity selected will reflect maintenance of the current status or level of functioning. The activity selected for the outcome should not deal with the etiology of the problem as stated in the nursing diagnosis but should address a lessening or elimination of the problem. For example:

Nursing Diagnosis: Pain related to movement, coughing and tissue trauma secondary to surgery.

Client Behavior: "Client rates pain as a 3 or less . . ." (deals with problem of pain) versus "Client demonstrates splinting of incision when coughing . . ." (deals with etiology of problem not directly with the pain).

The etiology of the pain problem above will be dealt with when the nurse selects interventions to meet the outcome of decreased pain. If the client can meet the outcome as written and still have no reduction in pain, then the outcome is incorrectly written. It is probably focused on the etiology part of the nursing diagnosis and is a nursing intervention rather than an outcome. In the example above, teaching the client to splint and support the incision before turning or coughing is an intervention to help meet the outcome of having the client rate the pain at 3 or less.

When writing an outcome statement, the word "client" or "patient" or the actual name of the person may be omitted since the outcome always refers to the client.

CLIENT BEHAVIOR = an observable activity the client will demonstrate at some time in the future showing improvement in the problem area

—(the client) will drink	(for a problem with hydration)
—(the client) will void	(for an elimination problem)
—decrease in (the client's) weight	(for a nutrition problem)

—(the client) will ambulate   (for a mobility problem)
—states signs of infection   (for a knowledge deficit diagnosis)

A caution about writing an outcome stating that the client will attend some type of class or meeting. Answer the question why do you want the client to attend this class or meeting? What outcome do you hope for? Unless the problem is social isolation or loneliness, this type of outcome statement is usually an intervention rather than an outcome. If the diagnosis is knowledge deficit, attending a class on the area of the deficit is not an outcome. It is an intervention. The client could attend the class and learn nothing and still meet this type of outcome. The real outcome would be for the client to state or demonstrate the knowledge or skill the nurse hoped was learned by attending the class.

CRITERION OF PERFORMANCE.   The criteria of performance is a stated level or standard for the client behavior stated in the outcome. This part of the outcome specifies a realistic improvement in functioning in the problem area by a stated time and will be used to determine if the outcome was satisfactorily achieved. The criterion clarifies and individualizes the outcome based on client's current abilities and realistic expectation for their level of functioning in the future. If the behavior selected for the outcome is to pass the course Nsg 101, is a grade of "D" an acceptable criterion for achievement or should the minimum criterion be set at the "C" level? Some outcomes identify the optimum level of recovery or functioning for a client after treatment and nursing care and often span days, weeks, or months. The time frame portion of the outcome statement is addressed further in this section and will affect the criterion selected for each outcome. The level of functioning a client can achieve this shift or this week may be very different from a long-term total recovery criterion. Consider the time frame when selecting the criterion. The shorter the time frame, the smaller the expected progress toward elimination of the problem.
    CRITERION OF ACCEPTABLE PERFORMANCE = the level at which the client will perform the behavior. How well? How far? How much?

—at least 500 ml of fluids
—250 ml of urine or more
—at least 5 lb
—the length of the hall and back
—without contamination of the syringe
—accurately and safely

CONDITIONS.   Sometimes the nurse sets outcomes with the client that require the use or presence of certain environmental conditions. Conditions can be thought of as specific aides that will facilitate the client performing a behavior at the level specified in the criteria portion of the outcome statement. Not all outcomes will have a condition. If the condition is essential to the performance of the behavior, then include it. If it is not essential, leave it out.

CONDITIONS = the circumstances, if necessary, under which the behavior will be performed

—with the use of a walker
—with the use of a wheelchair
—with the help of family
—with the use of medication
—while on oxygen
—on twice-daily insulin injections
—while on a PCA (patient controlled analgesia machine)

TIME FRAME.   The outcome statement includes a time or date to clarify how long it would realistically take for the client to reach the level of functioning stated in the criteria part of the outcome. This is based on nursing knowledge, experience, and knowledge of the individual client. The time frames stated in the outcome may be minutes, hours, days, weeks, or months. Intermediate outcomes may be achieved relatively sooner compared with long-term outcomes, which usually span the time it would take for most clients to achieve maximum recovery.

a. Intermediate outcomes.   Intermediate outcomes identify behavior a client can achieve fairly quickly, in a matter of hours, in an 8-hour shift or on a daily basis. Occasionally intermediate outcomes will involve weeks or months in a long-term care facility or in home health nursing where maximum recovery is expected to take months or years. Intermediate outcomes are especially appropriate to acute care settings such as hospitals where most clients stay only a few days and continue to recover at home or in a long-term care facility.

If a problem is diagnosed that tends to worsen with the passage of time, in terms of hours or days, intermediate outcomes are more appropriate than long-term or final outcomes to guide care. The nurse wants to see a change in client behavior soon; the problem cannot be allowed to continue until physical or psychological damage occurs. For example, the client who is unable to void following surgery cannot be left for 24 hours with a filling bladder. Extreme discomfort and possible damage to the bladder or kidneys could be the consequence. An intermediate outcome is identified for a client following surgery, such as "reestablishment of urinary elimination within 6 to 8 hours after surgery." If the client is unable to achieve this intermediate outcome, a catheter is often inserted to empty the bladder and prevent damage. Not all intermediate outcomes are written on a client's plan of care. Working toward outcomes is a way of thinking. Rather than thinking of separate tasks to accomplish this shift, such as bed bath, V.S., R.O.M. exercises, and meds, the nurse thinks "What can I realistically accomplish with this client in the next few hours to help lessen or eliminate the diagnosed problem?"

Some examples of intermediate outcomes are the following:

Respirations below 30 breaths/minute within 1 hour.
Return of bowel sounds within 12 hours postop.
Passing flatus within 24 hours postop.
Temperature to be below 102°F within 1 hour.
Pain to be rated as 4 or less within 30 minutes.
For the reader of this book: Completion of Chapter 4 in the next hour.

When learning to write outcomes, start with intermediate outcomes. A beginning nursing student is not with the same client for long periods of time. Students may care for a client for only a few hours. By writing intermediate outcomes involving the length of time with the client, the student will be able to give the needed nursing care and evaluate the results. By evaluating whether the intermediate outcome was met before leaving the client, students will gain skill in writing realistic outcomes and in giving nursing care to meet those goals.

Intermediate outcomes are often developed to help the nurse and the client gauge progress toward final outcomes. By achieving intermediate outcomes, the client is gradually advanced to the improved or optimum level of functioning identified in the final outcome. Achievement of intermediate outcomes provides repeated satisfaction for both the nurse and the client, serving as evidence of progress and guidance for the future. For example, the nurse and the client have identified an outcome of "weight loss of 80 pounds in 1 year." Progressive intermediate outcomes are identified to help the nurse and the client measure progress toward achievement of the eventual outcome. For example,

Weight of 210 pounds by February 7.
Weight of 208 pounds by February 14.
Weight of 206 pounds by February 21.

A series of intermediate outcomes that a person can realistically accomplish in a stated time period is much more rewarding than striving for one long-term outcome. The repeated reinforcement a person receives from meeting intermediate outcomes can keep an individual motivated to achieve a final outcome. If intermediate outcomes are not achieved, new nursing interventions can be tried, more realistic outcomes can be selected, or the nurse may reanalyze the data and diagnosis to make sure the problem is accurately identified, and important to the client.

Some other examples of intermediate outcomes leading to long-term outcomes are the following:

1. "I will finish reading this book before final exams" might be a long-term outcome for a student in nursing. This student might accomplish the long-term outcome by progressive intermediate outcomes of reading one chapter each week.

2. "Client will demonstrate full use of broken arm within 6 months." This client might accomplish the long-term outcome by progressively increasing the amount and range of muscle/joint exercises.

3. "Performance of self-care activities within 3 months of cerebral vascular accident (stroke)." Progressive intermediate outcomes might focus on accomplishment of one self-care activity a week until the client is able to perform all activities independently (final outcome).
   Week of 10/10: Feeds self by end of week.
   Week of 10/17: Brushing teeth by end of week.
   Week of 10/24: Performs personal hygiene by end of week.
   Week of 10/31: Meets own mobility needs by end of week.

b. Long-term or final outcomes.   Long-term outcomes give direction for nursing care over time. These outcomes can be thought of as an eventual destination, whereas progressive intermediate outcomes are a series of stops on the way to the final destination of optimum recovery. Intermediate and final outcomes are similar to a cross-country car trip. You plan to be in Florida by March 28th. To achieve that long-term outcome, you must be in Chicago by March 25th, and in Georgia by March 27th. These stops along the way are intermediate outcomes to assist the eventual achievement of the long-term outcome. Long-term outcomes try to identify the maximum level of functioning possible for a client with a particular nursing diagnosis. Consider the prognosis of the client's health problems, resources available, strengths and weakness of the client and family, and nursing care abilities of personnel who will be working with the client and family. If the client has an alteration in some function, the long-term outcome is to restore a normal pattern of functioning, if possible. If that is not possible, the outcome deals with establishing a maximum level of functioning for the alteration and assisting the client to adjust to this altered level of functioning. Some examples of long-term outcomes are the following:

> Reestablishment of client's usual bowel elimination patterns in 2 months.
> Reestablish normal voiding patterns by 5 days postop.
> Breastfeeding 10 to 15 minutes/breast, every 2 to 5 hours, within 2 weeks of delivery.
> Self-care of colostomy 1 month after surgery.
> Client to state no longer afraid of having severe pain during terminal illness from cancer after 1 week on IV morphine pump.
> For the reader of this book: Utilization of the nursing process to assess, diagnose, plan, implement, and evaluate the care of clients, following graduation from a school of nursing.

Some outcomes are designed to maintain a continuous level of functioning during the time the client is receiving nursing care. These outcomes are usually related to high risk rather than actual nursing diagnoses. They do not have a specified time for achievement but rather imply systematic assessment and evaluation for as long as the problem exists. These outcomes span several days to weeks or more. For example:

1. Client to report pain management techniques are adequate during hospitalization.
2. Client to report pain remains below 4 on a 1–10 scale during the postoperative period.
3. Skin integrity maintained during hospitalization.
4. Normal breath sounds maintained during postoperative period.
5. Maintenance of body weight between 135 and 140 pounds.

These outcomes would be evaluated periodically as part of the plan of care rather than having a set time or date for evaluation as with other outcomes discussed. For example (see outcomes above):

1. Assess pain every 3 to 4 hours.
2. Assess pain on 1–10 scale every 3 to 4 hours.
3. Assess skin integrity every 2 hours.
4. Assess breath sounds every 4 hours.
5. Assess body weight every morning.

These assessments would then be documented in the client's chart until the potential for the problem was eliminated.

The following examples combine these elements of client behavior, criteria of performance, time frame, and a condition, if necessary, to form outcome statements.

Guidelines for Writing Outcome Statements

When learning to write outcomes based on nursing diagnoses, consider the following criteria:

1. **For an actual nursing diagnosis, the outcome is a client behavior that demonstrates reduction or alleviation of the problem.** Start with the nursing diagnosis. What is the problem? If the nursing diagnosis is "Acute pain related to broken right arm as evidenced by client's report, crying and elevated pulse," the outcome will demonstrate alleviation or lessening of the pain (not healing of the arm). If the nursing diagnosis is "Constipation related to dehydration and use of analgesics with codeine," the outcome deals with bowel elimination patterns showing restoration of normal function (not improved hydration or limiting the amount of codeine). The following examples in Table 4-1 demonstrate the relationship between the nursing diagnosis and the outcome. A gen-

OUTCOME STATEMENTS

Client Behavior	+ Criteria	+ Time	+ Condition (if relevant)
Weight gain	of ½ ounce	every day until discharge	on 24 calorie/oz formula.
Weight gain	of ¼ ounce	every day until discharge	on breast-feeding with no supplement.
Self-injection	of correct insulin dose, using sterile technique	by November 4	using an autoinjector.
Maintenance of joint mobility	at current level	while on bed rest.	
Regain	15 lbs	in 2 months	on 2300 cal. diet and twice daily insulin injections.
Oral intake	of 500 ml	by 3 P.M.	without abdominal distention, nausea or vomiting.
Report pain reduced	at a level of 4 or less	during the first 24° postop	with Demerol 50–100 mg IM q3–4 hrs. prn.
Report pain reduced	at a level of 4 or less	during 24°–48° postop	with the use of oral analgesics q3–4 hrs. prn.
Will void	at least 300 cc	before bladder becomes distended.	
Will void	at least 200 cc	within 6 hours	after removal of Foley catheter.

TABLE 4-1   RELATIONSHIP OF THE DIAGNOSIS TO THE OUTCOMES

Nursing Diagnoses	*Outcomes*
Alteration in bowel elimination:	Reestablish normal bowel pattern by discharge:
*constipation related to dehydration and bed rest as evidenced by hard to pass stool and no BM for 5 days	○ bowel movement by 3 P.M. today following Fleet enema
•constipation related to dehydration and bed rest	○ bowel movement tomorrow without use of enema
supporting data: no BM for 5 days; reports stool hard to pass	
Alteration in comfort:	Report of negligible pain by discharge
*pain related to tissue trauma secondary to surgery as evidenced by rating pain as 8, elevated pulse and BP 136/72	○ pain reported at a level of 3 or less within the next hour
•pain related to tissue trauma secondary to surgery	○ pain reduced to a level of 3 or less during the next 24 hours with IM analgesics
supporting data: pulse 92, BP 136/72 pain rated as 8	○ pain reduced to a level of 3 or less after 48 hours postop with oral analgesic
Ineffective airway clearance:	Independent maintenance of clear airway by 3/8:
*ineffective airway clearance related to weakness and lowered level of consciousness as evidenced by inability to remove secretions from back of throat	○ airway free of tracheal mucus within the next ½ hour
•ineffective airway clearance related to weakness and lowered LOC.	○ productive cough by 12 hours
supporting data: generalized weakness; gurgling of mucus in throat; difficult to arouse; 86 years old; 1 hr postop	○ clear breath sounds in 24 hours

* = PES format (problem + etiology + signs/symptoms)

• = (problem + etiology format)

○ = intermediate outcomes

eral nursing diagnostic category from the NANDA list is presented first, with individualized diagnostic statements underneath. Two formats are used for the diagnostic statement of actual nursing diagnoses, the three-part statement and the two-part statement with supporting data underneath. A long-term outcome and one or more intermediate goals are identified for each diagnosis.

2. **For potential nursing diagnoses, the outcome is a client behavior that demonstrates maintenance of the current status of health or functioning.** If the potential nursing diagnosis is "Impaired skin integrity: high risk, related to casting of left leg," the outcome will demonstrate maintenance of intact skin (not healing of the leg). If the nursing diagnosis is "High risk for impaired thermoregulation related to newborn status," the outcome demonstrates maintenance of the newborn's temperature in the normal range.

3. **The outcome is realistic for the client's capabilities in the time span you designate in your outcome.** An outcome for a preterm baby weighing 4 pounds that stated, "Baby will weigh 8 pounds at the end of 1 week," would be unrealistic for this newborn. But if the outcome stated, "Baby will weigh 4 1/2 pounds in 7 days," the capabilities of the client have been considered and make the outcome more realistic and more likely to be achieved. Experience, professional literature, references, use of a Care Map®, and advice from other more experienced nurses will help the student learn what is realistic for clients with particular problems.

4. **The outcome is realistic for the nurse's level of skill and experience.** If the nursing diagnosis is dealing with a problem beyond the nurse's role, the best course of action is to refer the problem to the appropriate professional. A client with a nursing diagnosis of "Altered nutrition: less than body requirements related to refusal to eat hospital food as evidenced by 5 lb weight loss" is referred to a dietitian. A client with a nursing diagnosis of "Impaired verbal communication related to recent stroke as evidenced by inability to say any word except 'no,' " is referred to a speech therapist when the client's condition is sufficiently stable.

5. **The outcome is congruent with and supportive of other therapies.** This means that outcomes for the client do not contradict or interfere with the work of other professionals caring for the client. If the nursing diagnosis is "Urinary retention related to decreased urge, and perineal swelling as evidenced by residual urine volumes over 500 cc × 2," an intermediate outcome to have the client void 300 cc this shift would be in conflict with a medical order to leave the catheter in place for 12 hours if the second residual urine was more than 200 cc.

6. **Whenever possible the outcome is important and valued by the client, the nurses, and the physician.** If outcomes are important to clients, they will be more motivated to reach them. If nurses value the outcomes, they will be more likely to carry out the suggested plan of care. The physician's understanding and support of nursing outcomes will help to assure congruence with medical treatment. The outcomes also serve as a commu-

nication tool that keeps health team members informed of the client's progress.

7. **The outcome is an observable or measurable client behavior.** This means the nurse can see, hear, feel, or measure the client's response. Try to avoid words such as good, normal, adequate, and improved. These words mean different things to different people and tend to make the outcome unclear. There may be disagreement as to whether the outcome was achieved if words requiring a judgment are used in the outcome statement. Remember, the nurse cannot see a client "understanding," "feeling," or "knowing about."

Observable verbs

reports	eats	sleeps
walks	drinks	breathes
rates	voids	demonstrates

Observable Outcomes	Vague Outcomes
The client will walk the length of the hall unassisted by 2/5.	Increased ambulation or adequate leg strength
Client will gain ¼ lb each week until discharged.	Increased intake or good nutrition or promote weight gain

8. **Write outcomes in terms of client behavior, not nursing actions.**

Client Outcomes	Nursing Actions
The client will void by 6 P.M.	I will offer the client the urinal every 2 hours.
The client will safely bathe her baby before she is discharged.	I will show the client a baby bath before she is discharged.
The client's temperature will be up to 98°F within 1 hour.	I will put warm blankets and a heating pad on the client and recheck his temperature in 1 hour.

9. **Keep the outcome short.**
10. **Make the outcome specific.**
11. **Derive each outcome from only one nursing diagnosis.**
12. **Designate a specific time for achievement of each outcome.**

OUTCOMES: THE NEXT GENERATION

As mentioned in Chapter 2 (Assessment), the case management system is being widely adopted in the 1990s. One tool that has been developed is the CareMap® (Zander, 1991). Part of the CareMap® identifies the nursing diagnosis and related outcomes appropriate for approximately 75% of clients with a particular DRG. This tool is a preprinted form that specifies intermediate and final outcomes, achievable by hospital discharge, for clients admitted under a particular DRG category. It is based on the knowledge and clinical judgment of nurses and physicians who have collaborated to identify the progress in terms of outcomes that clients need to make to achieve maximum recovery in an efficient manner. The intermediate outcome and final outcomes identified in the CareMap® are considered standards of care and serve as guidelines for all health professionals caring for these clients. This tool is replacing the traditional nursing care plan in some clinical settings but includes all the components of the nursing process. (See Table 4-4 at the end of this chapter.) The diagnosis and related outcomes are the top half of the CareMap®.

PRACTICE EXERCISE

Pick out the correctly written outcomes. Identify what is wrong with the incorrectly written ones. The answers follow the exercise.

1. The client's hydration will improve.
2. The nurse will reduce the client's anxiety.
3. The client will know about infant feeding.
4. Improve muscle strength.
5. 3/5: The client will lose 6 lbs in 2 weeks.
6. The client will talk about her labor within 24 hours after delivery.
7. The decubitus ulcer (bedsore) will be healed by 2/5.
8. Verbalization of decreased pain within the next hour.
9. The client will express confidence in her ability to breast-feed her baby before discharge.
10. Turn and deep breathe the client every 2 hours.
11. Ankle edema will decrease.
12. The client will feel better by bedtime.
13. The client will ambulate.
14. Teach the client AROM (active range of motion) exercises.
15. The client's depression will improve.
16. The client will learn about good nutrition.
17. The client will understand the purpose of his medications before discharge.

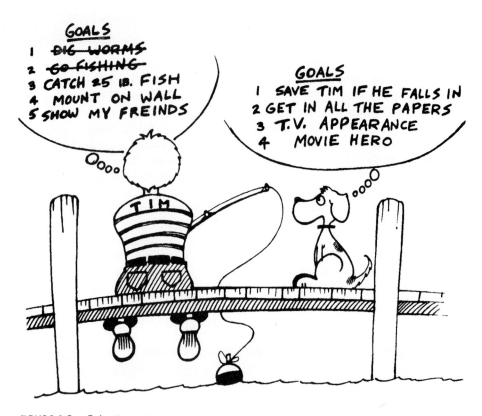

FIGURE 4-2.   Selecting outcomes.

18. The client's temperature will stay below 101°F during the next 24 hours.
19. The nursing student will understand the nursing process after reading this book.
20. The student will write a nursing diagnosis and final (long-term) outcome with two intermediate outcomes after finishing this chapter.

ANSWERS TO EXERCISE ON OUTCOME STATEMENTS

1. Not specific or observable. A better outcome would be:
   The client's intake will be 2500 cc every 24 hours.
   or
   The client will drink at least 75 cc each hour.
2. Not observable. This is a nurse behavior instead of client behavior. No time limit is set. A better outcome would be:

Verbalization of reduced anxiety about tomorrow's surgery by 10 P.M. tonight.

or

The client will discuss feelings related to biopsy by 3 P.M. today.

3. Not observable, no time limit. A better outcome would be:
States how to prepare formula by discharge.

or

Newborn regained birth weight on breast milk by 2-week checkup.

4. No subject, not specific, no criteria. A better outcome would be:
The client will lift his own weight using the bed trapeze by 2/5.

or

4/5: The client will lift equal amounts of weight in 3 months with his right and his left arm.

5. O.K.

6. O.K.

7. O.K.

8. Subject (the client) is assumed. Is any decrease in pain acceptable for achievement of this intermediate outcome? If pain goes from "unbearable" to "very severe," would you be satisfied? Would the client? Better outcome: Pain rated as 3 or less at the end of 1 hour.

9. O.K.

10. This is a nursing action, not an observable client behavior.

11. Not specific, no time limit. A better outcome would be:
Absence of edema of the ankle by tomorrow at 10 P.M.

or

Ankle will measure 10 inches in circumference or less by tomorrow at 8 A.M.

12. Not observable. A better outcome would be:
The client will state anxiety about being hospitalized has decreased by h.s.

13. No criteria. A better outcome would be:
The client will walk the length of the hall by date of discharge without use of a walker.

or

8/2: The client will walk from his bed to a chair in his room by tomorrow.

14. Nursing action instead of client behavior, no time limit. A better outcome would be:
The client will demonstrate AROM by 3 P.M. today.

or

The client will have equal motion in the right and left shoulder joint by time of discharge.

15. Too vague, not observable. A better outcome would be:
The client will sit in patient lounge for 15 minutes during this shift.

or

8/3: The client will get dressed and comb her hair tomorrow A.M.

16. Not observable. A better outcome would be:
(The client) Select a food from each of the four basic food groups for tonight's supper.
or
(The client) Plan a week's menu for a low-salt diet with the help of the dietitian before discharge.
17. Not observable. A better outcome would be:
The client will state the purpose of each of his medications before discharge.
or
By 4/7, the client will state route, dose, and time for each take-home medication.
18. O.K.
19. Not observable. A better outcome would be:
The nursing student will list the steps in the nursing process after reading this book.
or
The nursing student will write one nursing care plan after reading this book.
20. O.K.

PLANNING NURSING INTERVENTIONS

Nursing interventions are activities the nurse plans and implements to help a client achieve identified outcomes. By achieving these outcomes, the client will reduce or eliminate the diagnosed problems. Nursing interventions may be referred to in several ways: nursing actions, nursing strategies, nursing treatment plans, and nursing orders. This text will use all these terms to mean the same things. Some texts use the term nursing interventions to mean a general activity, such as "force fluids" and a nursing action or order then refers to a specific, individualized activity, such as "100 cc fluids q2h × next 24°." The nurse, using a problem-solving approach, selects activities to do with and for the client that are most likely to result in achievement of the outcome. There are many nursing interventions to choose from to help reduce a given problem. The nurse tries to select the best ones, based on the desired outcome, client abilities and preferences, available resources, nursing knowledge and experience, and protocols of the health care facility.

The planned nursing interventions are communicated to other nurses on the client's care plan to promote a consistent approach toward achievement of an outcome. Often the nurse who has the most information about the client and expertise in the particular problem areas diagnosed is the one who selects the most appropriate nursing interventions. The written care plan communicates this plan for outcome achievement to others who will provide 24-hour nursing care to the client. The nursing interventions written on the client's care plan are instructions for others to follow, since they may not have the knowledge of, or experience with, the client that the original nurse gained during the assessment phase.

Nursing interventions are similar to physician's orders since they specify a plan of care aimed at achieving an outcome. In order for others to follow a plan of care, it must be specific or the plan may be interpreted inappropriately. Interventions should identify:

—what is to be done
—when the activity is to be done; how often
—the duration for each intervention, when appropriate
—any preceding or follow-up activities
—the date interventions were selected
—the sequence in which nursing activities are to be performed, when one activity is dependent on or facilitated by a previous action
—signature or initials of the nurse writing the plan of care

When these things are identified by the professional nurse on a client's plan of nursing care, other nurses are held responsible and accountable to the client, nurse colleagues, and the health care facility for the prescribed care. Other nurses know to whom to direct questions regarding the client. They know to whom to direct feedback regarding client responses following the prescribed care. Physicians may seek out the nurse who wrote the plan of care for a client as the person most knowledgeable about that client's response to ordered treatments. All of this may seem somewhat threatening to the student in nursing who may feel unsure of abilities to identify accurate diagnoses, select appropriate outcomes, and choose nursing interventions most likely to achieve those outcomes. It is a learning process, but without both positive and negative feedback from other nurses who carry out the plan, students will not improve skills in planning client care.

> **NURSING INTERVENTIONS:**
> *Those specific activities the nurse plans and implements in order to help the client achieve an outcome.*

Types of Nursing Interventions

There are several broad categories of nursing interventions. Combining actions from several different groups is often the most effective plan. These groupings of nursing interventions include:

1. **Environmental management**—This aspect of nursing care involves establishing and maintaining a safe, therapeutic environment. A noisy, clut-

tered, stark environment is not the best atmosphere to promote rest and recovery. Attention to room order, opening and closing curtains for light, wall calendars showing the correct date, opening and reading mail, keeping the bed clean and straightened and the night stand accessible with needed personal articles are all activities that fall into this category. These activities may not require the expertise of a professional nurse, but it may be the nurse's responsibility to help with or delegate these activities. The client and family may be uneasy in a health care setting where no one attends to environmental management.

"Very few people ... have any idea of the exquisite cleanliness required in the sick room. ... The well have a curious habit of forgetting that what is to them but a trifling inconvenience, to be patiently "put up" with, is to the sick a source of suffering, delayed recovery, if not actually hastening death. The well are scarcely ever more than eight hours, at most, in the same room. Some change they can make, if only for a few minutes. ... But the sick man who never leaves his bed, who cannot change by any movement of his own his air, or his light, or his warmth; who cannot obtain quiet, or get out of the smoke, or the dust; he is really poisoned or depressed by what is to you the merest trifle."   p. 92

Florence Nightingale, *Notes On Nursing: What It Is and What It Is Not.* From an unabridged republication of the first American edition as published in 1860. (1969) New York: Dover Publications.

---

2. **Physician initiated and ordered interventions**—Based on the physician's diagnosis of the client's health problems, orders to assess client status, schedule tests, and provide treatments will be written by the physician in the client's chart. The nurse is expected to implement these orders. Implementation of these orders is still considered part of nursing interventions because the nurse individualizes the way the order is carried out based on the client's status at the time. The nurse often explains what is to be done and why. The nurse may give the client some choices within the scope of implementing the order. The timing of the implementation is often adjusted or designated by the professional nurse to fit in with constraints on personnel within the health care setting while still providing safety for the client and performance of the ordered activity. An example is IV therapy. The physician orders the type and amount of fluid to infuse and the rate. The nurse often does the venipuncture, sets up the IV system and keeps it running. The nurse assesses the client response frequently and may discontinue the infusion if problems develop. The nurse may refer the problem to a specially trained IV nurse to restart treatment. Based on other assessments of the client, the nurse may discuss with the physician

if IV therapy is required since the client is now drinking well with good bowel sounds.

3. **Nurse initiated and physician ordered interventions**—Based on the nurse's assessment of the client, and identification of problems, the nurse may request help from the physician in treatment. The nurse is not licensed to order certain treatments but recognizes when they may be needed. The nurse is requesting an intervention order from the physician to help reduce or treat the problem the nurse has identified. An order to catheterize a client unable to void may be written after the nurse notifies the physician of the problem, supporting data, and ineffective interventions implemented thus far. This type of intervention is most common when working with a collaborative problem rather than nursing diagnoses.

    Another example of this type of intervention occurs when the nurse collaborates with the physician regarding an order already written. The nurse may have identified a change in client status and is questioning whether an order should be implemented as written or whether the physician would like to change the order based on current client status and needs. For example, the physician may have written the order to begin clear liquids postoperatively and to discontinue the IV when the current bag has infused. The client is experiencing a variation from the normal postop course and is unable to take any fluids, is nauseated and vomiting, and has an increased pulse. To discontinue the IV at this point would not be prudent without updating the physician on the client's response postop. The nurse requests the physician's help, identifies the alteration in client status, and requests clarification of the original order.

    The physician frequently writes orders to be implemented only if the need arises (prn orders). The nurse then identifies if the problem develops, adapts the interventions to the client's status, implements the adapted order, and documents the client's response. This is the case when the physician writes prn orders for different forms of analgesia in a dosage range on a client. The nurse and the client determine need for the medication, intensity of pain, type of pain, and effectiveness of last analgesia, and the nurse selects the medication and dose most likely to meet the client's need for pain relief.

4. **Nurse initiated and ordered interventions**—These interventions are solely in the range of professional nursing. The nurse assesses the client, makes a nursing diagnosis, selects interventions, and implements those interventions or delegates implementation to other nursing personnel.

    Within this category are several forms of independent nursing interventions:
    a. health teaching
    b. health counseling to help clients make informed choices
    c. referrals to other nurses or health care professionals; transfer summaries to other stations, hospitals, or nursing homes; public health referrals; home health agency referrals

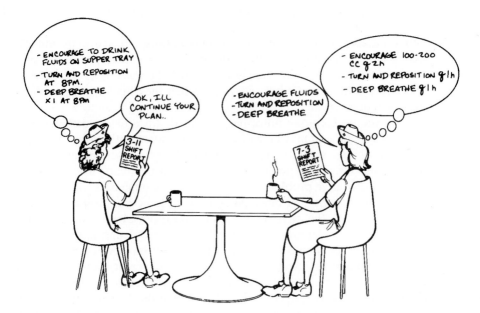

FIGURE 4-3.   Care plans ensure continuity of care when written in specific rather than general terms.

    d. specific nursing treatments to prevent problems or lessen current difficulties, such as ambulating, turning and repositioning, suctioning the airway, feedings, cleaning and dressing a wound, range of motion exercises, optimum nutrition

    e. providing support, comfort, and encouragement

    f. assessment of client status or response to treatments ordered by nursing, by physicians, or other health professionals

    g. discharge planning related to life-style changes, coping with health changes and medical treatments, setting priorities. Examples might include problem solving with a new diabetic client on how to fit blood glucose monitoring, insulin injections, and food intake into a job requiring frequent travel and eating in restaurants

    h. assistance with meeting basic needs/activities of daily living and ensuring safety.

Some examples of nursing interventions are the following:

INTERMEDIATE OUTCOME: Reestablish urinary elimination, with complete emptying of the bladder within 6 hours of removal of catheter.

—Interventions:

- Offer assistance to the bathroom for voiding every 2 hours
- Encourage fluids, 1 glass of juice, every hour
- Record intake and output for 24 hours

- Offer analgesics every 3 to 4 hours
- Provide privacy for voiding attempts
- Run water in bathroom for voiding attempts
- Encourage application of pressure over bladder during voiding attempts
- Encourage voiding attempt in sitz bath, tub bath, or shower if unable to void in 5 hours
- Assess bladder for emptying following voiding

Rationale for Nursing Interventions

Nursing actions are based on principles and knowledge integrated from previous nursing education and experience and from the behavioral and physical sciences. These principles identify the relationship between the nursing intervention and achievement of outcomes. Nursing actions are known to affect people in predictable ways and are chosen to help a client achieve these expected outcomes. For example, the effects of heat and cold applied to the skin are understood by the nurse. If the nurse wants to increase the blood flow to an area of the body as one way of promoting intermediate outcome achievement, a nursing intervention such as "warm packs to right arm, 20 minutes 4 times a day" might be chosen.

The first courses in many nursing programs involve the student in a study of fundamentals of nursing practice. These fundamentals courses provide the student with the rationale for the steps of various skills and procedures in addition to teaching the motor aspects of the skill or procedure. In order to safely adapt nursing care to new situations, new equipment, and changing technology, the nurse must understand the rationale behind the choice of nursing actions. Principles and theories related to sterile technique, for example, have remained constant as equipment and materials changed from reusable supplies to disposable. The nurse who understands the rationale behind sterile technique for various procedures is more able to adapt nursing care to a particular client using any variety of equipment and supplies available. Principles and theories from disciplines related to nursing, such as anatomy, physiology, microbiology, psychology, and sociology, blend with nursing knowledge and experience to form an integrated base of knowledge that guides the nurse in planning client care. While the nursing process involves an understanding of the rationale underlying nursing actions, it is not necessary to include this written rationale in documenting the care plan. However, the nursing process is incomplete and potentially unsafe unless nurses base their choices of nursing actions on appropriate rationale. Rationale for nursing actions are included in the various care plans in this text as a teaching tool. In clinical settings, writing rationales for nursing actions consumes much time and space and therefore is inappropriate.

The following example illustrates the principles and theories from various disciplines upon which selection of appropriate nursing actions are based.

NURSING DIAGNOSIS: Sleep pattern disturbance related to hospitalization, pain, and traction as evidenced by inability to fall asleep, reports of fatigue.

INTERMEDIATE OUTCOME: Improve nighttime sleep to at least 4 hours tonight.

LONG-TERM OUTCOME: Sleeping 6 hours/night by discharge without sleeping medication.

Nursing Interventions	Rationale
a. Obtain a sleep history	a. Provides baseline data from which to assess activities that promote or interfere with sleep
b. Assess for factors in the current environment that interfere with sleep and minimize if possible	b. Noise, heat, cold, too hard or soft a bed, roommates, lights, can all interfere with sleep
c. Offer pain medication at HS	c. Pain can interfere with sleep
d. Offer backrub at HS	d. Backrubs help to relax muscles and provide the client time to talk about any concerns; relaxation and decreased anxiety facilitate sleep
e. Help to reposition in traction	e. Good body alignment decreases strain on muscles and promotes comfort to facilitate sleep
f. Encourage good sleep hygiene ○ no caffeine after noon meal ○ limit cigarette smoking ○ offer light snack before bed ○ help to follow usual routine for hygiene, time to retire	 ○ caffeine is a stimulant ○ nicotine can stimulate CNS ○ foods high in protein and L-tryptophan (milk) promote sleep ○ normal habits from home are associated with a good sleeping pattern

Problem Solving and Selecting Interventions

How does a nurse choose the most appropriate interventions? Some nurses just seem to "know" what to do to help a client achieve an outcome. Others do things because "we have always done it this way." Still others rely on a standard care plan designed for all clients with a similar problem to tell them what to do. Where does a student begin? Nursing students do not base care on intuition. They have to learn how to be effective nurses. That means applying the skills of problem solving to a particular client's health problems and the environment in which nursing care is to be given. The following suggestions may be helpful when selecting interventions:

1. Review the nursing diagnosis so the problem and etiology of the problem is clear. For *actual problems*, try to reduce or eliminate the problem and the cause (etiology) of the problem. If the cause cannot be reduced or eliminated, select interventions to minimize or eliminate the problematic signs and symptoms. For *high-risk problems*, select interventions which reduce or eliminate the risk factors. If this is not possible, select interventions to prevent the problem from developing, delay its development, or reduce the severity of the problem when it does develop. For example, insulin dependent diabetics are at risk for tissue damage in the legs and feet. Teaching good foot care and maintenance of blood glucose levels as close to normal as possible may delay or prevent this complication or make it less severe and more easily treated.

2. Examine the intermediate and final outcomes so you know where you're going and the steps to get there.

3. Consider all possible nursing activities that might help the client achieve the outcome:
    —changes in the environment
    —activities for the client and family to perform independently
    —activities to perform with the client
    —activities to perform for the client
    —assistance from other health care professionals
    —involvement of the client's friends and family
    —changes in the nurse (increased knowledge and skill)

4. Use standard care plans as guidelines for developing and planning a client's nursing care. Standard client's care plans may be available to you on preprinted forms that will fit in a Kardex care plan or in the chart. These standards provide the nurse with general guidelines for clients with particular medical diagnoses, diagnostic studies, or nursing diagnoses. They identify areas for assessment, possible client problems to anticipate, and suggested outcomes and nursing interventions. They provide the student and the nurse with another resource for planning nursing interventions. These standard care plans do not replace the individualized care plan developed by the nurse. Based on the knowledge about an individual client, the medical management of health problems, the health care setting, and client and family preferences and concerns, the nurse will: fill out the etiology and signs and symptoms of the diagnosis, select and individualize outcomes from a list of possible outcomes, delete inappropriate interventions, add new interventions, and individualize general interventions. These plans save the nurse time in rewriting common nursing interventions but do not replace the process of planning individualized care. See Table 4-2.

5. Use the client and the client's family as a source of possible nursing interventions. Clients and their families may have many good suggestions for activities the client can perform, with or without nursing assistance, to achieve a certain outcome, based on the client's past experiences and personal preferences. The nurse then uses personal knowledge and expe-

TABLE 4-2   NURSING DIAGNOSIS STANDARD OF CARE   ADDRESSOGRAPH

Pain related to _____

("A state in which an individual experiences and reports the presence of severe discomfort or an uncomfortable sensation," NANDA, 1992)
Client Characteristics: _____

Client Outcome Standards:
___ Verbalization that pain has been eliminated or decreased to a level of
   _____ on a scale of 1–10 by _____.
                     during _____.
___ Evaluation: _____
___ Reduction in values of vital signs: P, R, BP, toward normal range
   by _____.
___ Evaluation: _____
Other: _____
___ Evaluation: _____

Nursing Intervention Standards:
  1.   Assess pain and related factors.
       a. intensity (1–10) _____
       b. duration _____
       c. character (sharp, dull, shooting, burning) _____
       d. location _____
       e. precipitated by _____
  2.   Assess for effectiveness of previous pain relief interventions.
       a. previous medication (drug, dose, route, effectiveness on 1–10) ____
          _____
       b. other helpful measures: _____
          _____
  3.   Offer _____ (analgesic ordered by MD) q _____ prn.
  4.   Encourage use of analgesics before _____
       (pain precipitating activity) at _____ am/pm or _____
  5.   Offer relaxation techniques: slow relaxed breathing _____
                               music _____
                               backrub _____
                               heat _____
  6.   Assist with repositioning as needed q _____
  7.   Encourage use of distracting stimuli: radio, TV, other: _____
       effleurage/skin stroking _____

Developed by _____ date: _____
Evaluated by _____ date: _____
Reviewed/Updated by _____ date: _____

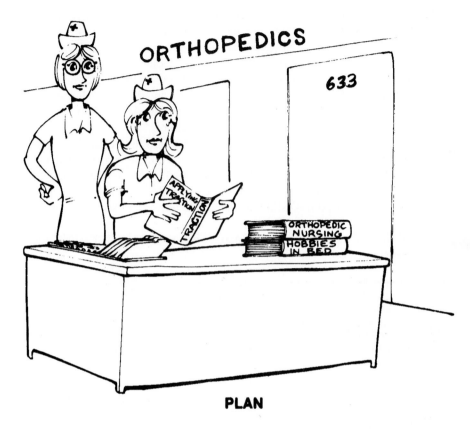

FIGURE 4-4. Use resources and more experienced nurses for help in selecting interventions.

rience to incorporate some of these suggestions into a plan of care. This collaboration helps to involve clients and their families in planning and implementing the type of nursing care they receive. By using the client and family to help plan nursing interventions, the nurse considers client preferences, which usually leads to more effective interventions.

6. Use resources, such as nursing fundamentals texts, medical-surgical nursing texts, and current journal articles. Use the policy and procedure manual on the clinical setting for information on what is to be done and how to do it in a particular setting.

7. Consider the advantages and disadvantages of possible nursing interventions and select those that meet the following criteria:

• **Nursing actions must be safe for the client.** Application of heat to the skin will stimulate circulation, but excessive heat will burn. Nursing actions using heat must ensure that the client is not burned. Exercising a client's muscles and joints can be very beneficial; however, if muscles and joints are forced beyond the point of resistance or pain, the nurse can cause injuries.

- **Nursing actions must be congruent with other therapies.** For example, nursing actions must be selected within the safety range ordered by the physician. If the medical order reads "Aspirin (ASA), 2 tablets, q4h, prn," nursing actions cannot plan the administration of aspirin every 2 hours. If the physical therapist is instructing the client in the use of a walker, the nurse should also use a walker in ambulating the client.
- **Nursing actions selected are most likely to develop the behavior described in the outcome.** There may be many different nursing actions that would accomplish the same outcome. The nurse attempts to give the client practice in the specific behavior stated in the outcome. For example:
  - NURSING DIAGNOSIS: Pain related to movement secondary to bone cancer.
  - OUTCOME: Verbalization of pain as less than 3 on a 1–10 scale during hospitalization.

Nursing Actions/Interventions	
May Achieve Outcome	*More Likely to Achieve Outcome*
a. Offer prescribed pain medication q3–4h prn	a. Assess client's pain, timing, duration, intensity, and related activities, q3–4h
	b. Administer analgesic ½ hour before physical therapy
	c. Administer analgesic q3h while awake
	d. Assess client's current methods of dealing with pain and support if possible
	e. Discuss and practice alternate pain relief measures with client by March 1
	(1) Relaxation
	(2) Alternative sensory stimulation
	—music
	—tactile (massage, effleurage, menthol rubs, vibrators)
	—heat/cold
	—movies, TV, reading
	(3) Breathing techniques
	f. Discuss self-medication for pain, by March 3

Nursing Actions/Interventions

May Achieve Outcome	*More Likely to Achieve Outcome*
	g. Discuss effectiveness of pain relief measures with physician and client
	h. Encourage use of pain relief measures when discomfort *begins* rather than after it is intense

- **Nursing actions are realistic:**
  - —for the client. Consider age, physical strength, disease, willingness to change behavior, resources.
  - —for the number of hospital staff. Will enough people consistently be available to carry out the nursing actions?
  - —for the experience and ability of available staff. If most of the staff are unfamiliar with the nursing actions you are suggesting or disagree with it, there is a high probability they will not be carried out.
  - —for available equipment. If your nursing actions include the use of any equipment, it should be readily available and the hospital staff should be familiar with its use.
- **Nursing actions consider meeting lower level survival needs before higher level needs.** For example, the following sequence of nursing actions deals with the current need of pain avoidance before asking the client to deal with high-risk problems.
  - NURSING DIAGNOSIS: High risk for ineffective breathing pattern related to general anesthesia, postop pain.
  - OUTCOME: Normal respiratory rate and lung sounds by 2nd day postop.
  - NURSING INTERVENTIONS:
    a. Reduce pain to a level of 4 or less on a 1–10 scale
    b. Explain the potential problem and outcome to client.
    c. Explain preventive function of the following activities.
      (1) Turning, coughing, and deep breathing at least every 2 hours.
      (2) Early ambulation.
      (3) Use of deep-breathing device, q1 h
    d. Explain ways to minimize discomfort during turning and coughing; splinting, analgesics.
    e. Offer pain medication 1/2 hour prior to ambulating.
    f. Assist client to:
      (1) TCH q2 h × 24 h
      (2) Ambulate q.i.d. starting first postop day.
      (3) Deep breath q1 h while awake × 24 h.
    g. Assess lung sounds before and after TCH sessions.

- **Whenever possible, nursing actions should be important to the client and compatible with personal goals and values.** The client should understand how the nursing actions will result in achievement of the outcome. For example, a man may refuse to do arm and hand exercises because he does not think they are important. If the nursing actions encourage the client to do activities such as shaving, combing his hair, brushing his teeth, and feeding himself, the arms and hands will still receive the desired exercise. The difference is that the client values being able to do these self-care activities and can see that they are part of his recovery.

Client Teaching: An Intervention Strategy

If the nurse assesses a client and makes a nursing diagnosis with an etiology or risk factors related to a knowledge or performance deficit, a teaching plan will most likely comprise a large portion of the activity in the planning phase of the nursing process. Many plans of care include a teaching component for each outcome as the nurse explains what is to be done and why. One of the standards by JCAHO for hospital accreditation states that: "Throughout the patient's stay, the patient and, as appropriate, his/her significant other(s) receive education specific to the patient's health care needs." (JCAHO, 1992). Unrealistic fears of a medical procedure and incorrectly taking prescribed medications are examples of problems that could be caused by the client's belief in erroneous information. Clients with newly diagnosed medical problems are frequently confronted with knowledge deficits concerning the implications of their medical diagnosis and the effect it may have on their life-style. Clients taking on new roles, such as parenting, are frequently concerned about their lack of knowledge and skill in newborn care. Prenatal classes such as Lamaze and CEA will anticipate these learning needs and identify specific areas of newborn care that prospective parents would like to discuss in class. Nursing follow-through in the hospital, after delivery, builds on this information and gives the parents actual practice in caring for their newborn. Similarly, preoperative and postoperative teaching is based on a nursing diagnosis of inadequate knowledge of the surgical experience, complications, and preventive measures. Preoperative teaching is also based on research indicating that an educated client, knowing what will happen during a procedure, will often experience less pain and anxiety than an unprepared client. The nursing diagnosis, again, would relate to inadequate or incorrect information about a particular procedure or surgery.

In applying the nursing process to the formulation of a teaching plan, the nurse follows a logical sequence of problem solving. First, the knowledge deficit is identified based on data obtained during the assessment phase of the nursing process. A learning outcome is then chosen. Next, a plan is developed to teach the skill or information to the client and family, as appropriate.

For example:

1. NURSING DIAGNOSIS: Knowledge and skill deficit in taking newborn rectal temperature related to first-time parenting.

[This diagnosis might be written in an alternate form identifying inadequate knowledge and skill as the cause of a potential problem; "High risk for altered health maintenance related to lack of knowledge and skill in newborn temperature assessment."]

OUTCOME: Take an accurate rectal temperature on her newborn before discharge, on 3/5.

NURSING INTERVENTIONS (Teaching Plan):

1. Discuss when to take baby's temperature; signs and symptoms indicating illness.
2. Demonstrate how to take rectal temperatures on newborns, 3/4.
3. Explain safety precautions and when to notify physician for fevers, 3/4.
4. Provide reinforced practice in taking her newborn's temperature, 3/4.

2. NURSING DIAGNOSIS: Knowledge deficit in taking medications related to forgetting and not reading directions.

[This diagnosis might be written in an alternate form identifying the problem as caused by inadequate knowledge; "High risk for injury related to lack of knowledge of medications and administration."]

OUTCOME: Demonstrate correct self-administration of medication by 11/3.

NURSING INTERVENTIONS:

1. Check that client can read all labels on medications, 11/1.
2. Discuss with the client how to safely take each medication (drug, dose, time, route), 11/1.
3. Provide a clear set of directions in written form regarding medications, 11/1.
4. Supervise client in hospital with self-administration of prescribed medications, 11/1, 11/2.

When clients learn specific motor skills, the outcome selected has a very direct relationship to the diagnosed knowledge or performance deficit. The teaching plan and eventually the evaluation of the client's ability to perform the skill are usually equally specific. When teaching motor skills, follow the steps of the nursing process:

1. Assess current knowledge and skill ability (ASSESS)
2. Identify knowledge deficits (MAKE NURSING DIAGNOSIS)
   —Inadequate skill in performance of . . .
   —Knowledge deficit in area of . . .
   —High risk for (specify problem) related to lack of knowledge and/or skill in area of . . .
3. Identify the specific behavior the client will perform based on the diagnosed learning need (PLAN OUTCOMES).
4. Teach the specific behavior to the client (IMPLEMENT).

5. Evaluate the client's ability to perform the specific behavior (EVALUATE).

Evaluating client learning may be difficult if observable behaviors are not identified as outcomes during the planning phase. When a client is developing an understanding of broader concepts or improving cognitive skills, the nurse's teaching plan cannot focus on one specific behavior as evidence of this broader understanding. For example, if the diagnosis relates to inadequate knowledge of infant care, an outcome dealing with the isolated behavior of diapering does not provide support for the assumption that the parent is competent in infant care. In this case, the method the nurse may use is the identification of one long-term learning outcome and then identification of subsequent several intermediate outcomes that build toward the long-term outcome. The long-term outcome may be more difficult to state in behavioral terms. The examples of intermediate outcomes should be stated as observable or measurable behaviors. The teaching plan is then directed at the discharge outcome by achieving the intermediate outcomes.

Example 1:
NURSING DIAGNOSIS: Knowledge and skill deficit of newborn care related to new parent role.
LONG-TERM OUTCOME: Parents will safely care for newborn by time of discharge from hospital, on 11/3.
INTERMEDIATE OUTCOMES:
1. Demonstrate bathing their newborn, 11/2.
2. Safely take a rectal temperature on newborn, 11/2.
3. Demonstrate cord care for umbilical stump, 11/2.
4. Breast-feeding: 10–15 minutes per breast q2–5 h, by 11/3.
5. Transport newborn home from hospital in infant car seat, 11/3.

TEACHING PLAN: Nursing Interventions
1. Assess readiness for learning infant care (comfort level, fatigue, personal priority needs).
2. Discuss various aspects of infant care: feeding, hygiene, safety, growth and development, behavior.
3. Demonstrate specific infant care skills and provide practice for parents with positive reinforcement.
4. Assist in initiation of breast-feeding and provide specific information on the skill.
5. Provide resources for parents after discharge (people to call when questions or problems arise).
6. Follow-up phone call to answer questions 2–3 days postdischarge.

Example 2:
NURSING DIAGNOSIS: High risk for failure in Nursing 101 related to lack of knowledge of the nursing process as evidenced by 2 correct out of 15 points on the unit test.
LONG-TERM OUTCOME: Student will pass Nursing 101 with a grade of "C" or better by the end of the course.

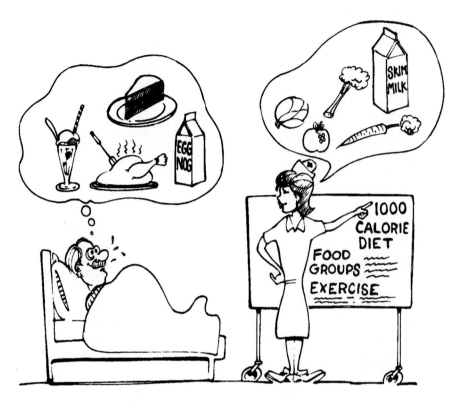

FIGURE 4-5.   A good teaching plan does not always guarantee that client learning will occur.

INTERMEDIATE OUTCOMES:
1.   Identify five phases of the nursing process, 3/1.
2.   Explain nursing diagnosis and how it differs from medical diagnosis, 3/5.
3.   Write three nursing diagnoses from a data base, 3/10.
4.   Write three nursing outcomes showing observable client behavior, and criteria of performance, 3/20.
5.   Write three sets of nursing interventions to help a client achieve three different outcomes by 4/1.
6.   Evaluate achievement of outcomes and review care plan by 4/10.

TEACHING PLAN: Nursing Interventions
1.   Assess readiness to learn; strengths and interfering factors.
2.   Discuss ways to reduce or eliminate factors interfering with learning.
3.   Discuss rationale for using the nursing process.
4.   Explain, briefly, the relationship between the nursing process, client care, and passing Nsg 101.
5.   Assign readings on nursing process.
6.   Demonstrate application of nursing process on a hypothetical client's data base.
7.   Use practice exercises for writing nursing diagnoses, client outcomes, and planning actions.

8. Written student assignment: Develop a care plan on four assigned hospital clients showing assessment, diagnosis, planning, implementation, and evaluation.
9. Review and critique other students' care plans.

There are several things to consider when developing a teaching plan. Learning is enhanced by using principles of teaching-learning. It is especially important to assess the client's readiness to learn. An illness, medical problem, or treatment may greatly interfere with learning, particularly in the acute

Common Components of a Teaching Plan	Rationale and Scientific Principles
1. Setting a learning outcome with the client.	1. Clarification of desired learning outcomes will guide teaching methods and may serve as a motivating function for the learner.
2. Assessing client's readiness to learn. a. motivation–recognizes knowledge deficit b. illness/medical problem c. medication/pain d. level of consciousness e. anxiety level f. fatigue	2. A person learns more effectively when the learning experience has personal relevance. A person learns more effectively when a need to learn is perceived. Unmet physical or psychosocial needs such as anxiety, pain, and fatigue have a negative effect on attention, retention, and ability to learn.
3. Assess client's current knowledge and motor skill ability. 4. Begin teaching at the client's current level of understanding or skill performance.	3., 4. Teaching that moves from simple to complex will help to ensure understanding. Simple and complex are relative terms and have meaning only in relationship to the learner's current level of understanding or performance.
5. Provide the client with an opportunity to practice motor skills after a demonstration. 6. Reinforce client's efforts to learn whenever possible.	5., 6. An active learner learns and retains more than a passive learner. Practice with feedback and positive reinforcement leads to improved performance and continuance of reinforced behavior.

A nurse promotes readiness to learn ...

. . . . I was working in the obstetrical unit of a university hospital. A baby had been born a few days ago with a cleft lip and palate. The mother had refused to see or hold the baby since delivery. She stayed in her room, cried frequently, and slept off and on during the day. The staff was getting quite fed up with her since the baby was healthy in every other way and she was supposed to take the baby home tomorrow. She had refused the information from the doctor on cleft lip and palate. We had delayed all efforts at teaching infant care based on her refusal to do anything with the baby. She was not ready to learn, but the reality of the hospital setting said she would be discharged with that baby tomorrow, ready or not. The problems of dysfunctional grieving, potential for altered parenting, and even potential for physical harm to the baby were all running through my mind in addition to the knowledge and skill deficit problem. I went in the room and she pulled the covers over her head and said "Go away." "Great start," I thought. "This is going to be a terrific shift!" As I sat down in a chair next to her, I was desperately trying to think of what to do. As honestly as I could, I shared my concerns and frustrations as the nurse for her and her baby. I also wanted her to know I wasn't condemning her or telling her she shouldn't feel the way she felt. "I'm so sorry about your baby, and I know you're very upset. You and the baby are supposed to go home tomorrow and I'm worried because I don't feel like you are ready." I told her what kind of teaching and hands-on care most new mothers are given in the hospital and how they often are still apprehensive about going home. I told her I didn't know how she was feeling or even if she was willing to care for the baby at home. "Your baby is eating very well, acting like all the other babies, crying, sleeping, stooling, and voiding." I was trying to point out what was normal about her baby. After a few moments of silence, I asked the new mother if I could feed her baby in her room because the baby was acting hungry when I left the nursery. The mother agreed, and I held and fed the baby. As I was doing this she reached out and touched the baby's feet and hands and commented on how perfectly they were formed. As I was leaving the room with the baby after the feeding, she asked me to bring her the information on cleft lip and palate that the doctor said he would leave at the nurse's station.

phase of an illness. Medications, fatigue, anxiety, pain, or hunger may all block effective learning. Grief over unexpected, negatively evaluated outcomes related to treatment, medical diagnosis, life-style changes, body changes or prognosis will often delay the desire for learning by the client. For example, the client who finally begins to look at her colostomy stoma and asks some questions about it, may be ready to listen to some information, while a few days ago she was unwilling to even acknowledge the presence of the colostomy as part of her body. Teaching should be delayed until some of these obstacles have been lessened or eliminated. The nurse also assesses the client's previous knowledge and skills, building on this prior base. Begin at the level of client and family understanding using language understandable to the client. Individualizing the teaching approach may also lead to improved client learning. The following principles support these common nursing interventions as part of a teaching plan.

Classification of Nursing Interventions

A research team at the University of Iowa began work in May of 1987 to develop a classification system for nursing interventions. This group is developing "a taxonomy (a classification system) of nursing interventions to include all direct care treatments that nurses perform on behalf of patients" (Bulechek and McCloskey, 1992, p. 290). They are using the definition of interventions from NANDA's eighth conference: "A nursing intervention is any direct care treatment that a nurse performs on behalf of a client. These treatments include nurse-initiated treatments resulting from nursing diagnoses, physician-initiated treatments resulting from medical diagnoses, and performance of the daily essential functions for the client who cannot do these" (Bulechek & McCloskey, in Carroll-Johnson, 1992). An excerpt from their early work is exemplified here in the area of pain management interventions. This particular grouping was chosen for inclusion in this chapter to make the nursing student aware of the Iowa group's work and because of the universality of interventions related to pain management in most clinical facilities where students will be practicing. See Tables 4-3 and 4-4.

NURSING INTERVENTIONS: THE NEXT GENERATION

In the case management model of health care delivery, a tool called *critical pathways* has evolved. This tool specifies which nursing interventions to implement and when to do them for all clients with a particular DRG. Both the critical nursing and medical interventions are usually included on the critical path tool. These actions have been identified by expert nursing clinicians, staff nurses, and physicians as the most effective actions to help clients meet preselected outcomes. For example, on the day of surgery the critical path may direct the nurse to stand the client at the bedside the evening of surgery. The next day the critical path would direct the nurse to ambulate the client in the hall, TID. All of these interventions would be aimed at meeting the discharge outcome of: "Ambulates unassisted with no dizziness by discharge." These

TABLE 4-3   TEN INTERVENTION LABELS RELATED TO PAIN: DEFINITIONS

Intervention	Definition
Pain Management	The alleviation of pain or a reduction in pain to a level of comfort that is acceptable to the patient.
Analgesic Administration	Use of pharmacologic agents to reduce or eliminate pain.
Environmental Management: Comfort	Manipulation of the patient's surroundings for promotion of optimal comfort.
Cutaneous Stimulation	Stimulation of the skin and underlying tissues for the purpose of decreasing undesirable signs and symptoms such as pain, muscle spasm, or inflammation.
Heat/Cold Application	Stimulation of the skin and underlying tissues with heat or cold for the purpose of decreasing pain, muscle spasms or inflammation.
Simple Massage	Stimulation of the skin and underlying tissues with varying degrees of hand pressure to decrease pain, produce relaxation and/or improve circulation.
Transcutaneous Electrical Nerve Stimulation (TENS)	Stimulation of skin and underlying tissues with controlled, low voltage electrical vibration via electrodes.
Distraction	Purposeful focusing of attention away from undesirable sensations.
Simple Guided Imagery	The purposeful use of imagination to achieve relaxation and/or direct attention away from undesirable sensations.
Simple Relaxation Therapy	Use of techniques to encourage and elicit relaxation for the purpose of decreasing undesirable signs and symptoms such as pain, muscle tension, or anxiety.

Adapted from Herr, K. & Mobily, P. (1992). Interventions related to pain. *Nursing Clinics of North America,* 27(2), 347–369.

interventions serve as minimum standards of practice: they define the process (actions) most likely to yield the desired outcomes. As mentioned earlier, these interventions are designed to serve as guidelines for caring for approximately 75% of clients with a particular DRG admission. However, each individual client will need the nurse to individualize these standard interventions for maximum effectiveness. Some interventions may need to be modified,

TABLE 4-4   ANALGESIC ADMINISTRATION

DEFINITION: Use of pharmacologic agents to reduce or eliminate pain

---

ACTIVITIES:

Determine pain location, characteristics, quality, and severity prior to medicating patient

Check medical order for drug, dose, and frequency of analgesic prescribed

Check history for drug allergies

Evaluate the patient's ability to participate in selection of analgesic, route, dose, and involve the patient as appropriate

Choose the appropriate analgesic, or combination of analgesics when more than one is prescribed

Determine analgesic selections (narcotic, non-narcotic, NSAID) based on type and severity of pain

Determine the preferred analgesic, route of administration, and dosage to achieve optimal analgesia

Choose the IV route, rather than IM, for frequent pain medication injections when possible

Monitor vital signs before and after administering narcotic analgesics with first time dose or if unusual signs are noted

Attend to comfort needs and other activities that assist relaxation to facilitate response to analgesia

Administer analgesics around-the-clock to prevent peaks and troughs of analgesia, especially with severe pain

Set positive expectations regarding the effectiveness of analgesics to optimize patient response

Administer adjuvant analgesics and/or medications when needed to potentiate analgesia

Consider use of continuous infusion either alone or in conjunction with bolus opioids to maintain serum levels

Institute safety precautions for those receiving narcotic analgesics as appropriate

Instruct to request PRN pain medication before the pain is severe

Inform the individual that with narcotic administration drowsiness sometimes occurs the first 2 to 3 days and then subsides

Correct misconceptions/myths patient or family members may hold regarding analgesics, particularly opioids (i.e., addiction, risks of overdose)

Evaluate the effectiveness of analgesic at regular frequent intervals following each administration, but especially after the initial doses, also observing for any signs and symptoms of untoward effects (e.g., respiratory depression, nausea and vomiting, dry mouth, constipation)

Document response to analgesic and any untoward effects

Evaluate and document level of sedation for patients receiving opioids

Implement actions to decrease untoward effects of analgesics (such as
   constipation, gastric irritation)
Collaborate with the physician if drug, dose, route of administration, or
   interval changes are indicated, making specific recommendations based on
   equianalgesic principles
Teach about the use of analgesics, strategies to decrease side effects, and
   expectations for involvement in decisions about pain relief

some interventions may need to be added, and some may be inappropriate
for a particular client. The time line may need to be altered for an individual
client who is progressing ahead of or behind the expected course. Another
tool, the CareMap,® includes the critical path in addition to the nursing diagnoses and intermediate and discharge outcomes. A key component of the
CareMap® is a separate sheet called a variance record for documenting the
changes a nurse makes while implementing the standard interventions with a
particular client. The variance record is the form on which the nurse records
why the standard intervention or time frame had to be altered and what action
or time frame replaced the original. Interventions the nurse selects to try to
get the client back on track and on schedule are also documented on the
variance sheet. Later these can be used to adapt the standard critical path
component of the CareMap® to make it more applicable, realistic, and effective. See Table 4-5 for an example of a student learning map based on the
concept of a CareMap®. Table 4-6 is an actual CareMap® developed for clients
with congestive heart failure.

SUMMARY

During the planning phase of the nursing process, the nurse and the client set
priorities among the identified problems, establish outcomes showing reduction, prevention or elimination of the problem, and plan interventions to
achieve these outcomes. An outcome is the desired behavioral change in the
client following nursing care. For actual nursing diagnoses, the outcomes identify client behavior demonstrating a lessening or elimination of the problem.
For high-risk nursing diagnoses, the outcomes demonstrate that clients are
maintaining the current level of functioning or preventing the problem from
developing. Outcomes give direction to nursing actions as do the nursing diagnoses. Longer-term outcomes, also called final outcomes or discharge
outcomes, demonstrate the maximum level of functioning for the client or

TABLE 4-5   LEARNING MAP   DRG CATEGORY—FIRST YEAR NURSING STUDENT 3RD QUARTER

Problems (Nursing dx.)	Time Line →				
	Day 1	Day 2	Day 3	Day 4	Day 5
	Intermediate Outcomes				Final Outcome
1) Knowledge deficit in IV meds and IV therapy	States principles of gravity flow IV system		States S & S of IV therapy complications and corrective nursing actions		Achieves 85% or higher on IV theory test
2) Skill deficit in IV meds & IV therapy	Sets up IV using new bag/tubing to run at 125cc/hr without contamination		Sets up IV med. piggyback to run at 100cc/hr without contamination in lab (day 3),	In clinical (day 4)	Achieves 90% or higher with no contamination on IV skills test
3) Injury: High risk related to learning skills of IV therapy	Injury-free during IV practice in lab				Injury-free during IV therapy in clinical setting

Critical Path—Student tasks (*Nursing Interventions*)	*Day 1*	*Day 2*	*Day 3*	*Day 4*	*Day 5*
	Attend lab/class	Attend lab/class	Attend clinical	Attend clinical	Take IV Theory test
	Do textbook reading	Do textbook reading	Observe client's IV system	Review theory content	Take IV Lab test
	Chs. 12, 13 Find a partner to practice I.V. set-up with	Ch. 14 Lab practice with partner —Using heparin lock —Regulating flow	Look up IV meds in drug book	Give IV med to client with instructor	
	Practice in lab with partner —spiking bag —filling tubing —attaching needle	Practice all skills with feedback from lab instructor	Assess client for complications	Observe IV nurse on rounds for 2 hours	
	Review math to calculate flow rates		Observe staff nurse give IV med	Get 6 hrs of sleep	

TABLE 4-6 CAREMAP™: CONGESTIVE HEART FAILURE

	Day 1 ER 1–4 hours	Day 1 Floor Telemetry or CCU 6–24 hours	Day 2 Floor	Day 3 Floor	Day 4 Floor	Day 5 Floor	Day 6 Floor
Location							
			Benchmark Quality Criteria				
Problem			*Diagnoses (1–7) and Outcomes*				
1) Alteration in gas exchange/ perfusion and fluid balance due to decreased cardiac output, excess fluid volume	Reduced pain from admission or pain free Uses pain scale O_2 sat. improved over admission baseline on O_2 therapy	Respirations equal to or less than on admission	O_2 sat = 90 Resp 20–22 Vital signs stable Crackles at lung bases Mild shortness of breath with activity	Does not require O_2 Vital signs stable Crackles at base Respirations 20–22 Mild shortness of breath with activity	Does not require O_2 (O_2 sat. on room air 90%) Vital signs stable Crackles at base Respirations 20–22 Completes activities with no increase in respirations No edema	Can lie in bed at baseline position Chest X-ray clear or at baseline	No dyspnea
2) Potential for shock	No signs/symptoms of shock	No signs/symptoms of shock	No signs/symptoms of shock	No signs/symptoms of shock Normal lab values	No signs/ symptoms of shock	No signs/ symptoms of shock	No signs/ symptoms of shock

Diagnosis							
3) Potential for consequences of immobility and decreased activity: skin breakdown DVT	No redness at pressure points / No falls	No redness at pressure points / No falls	Tolerates chair, washing, eating, and toileting	Has bowel movement / Up in room and bathroom with assist	Up ad lib for short periods	Activity increased to level used at home without shortness of breath	Activity increased to level used at home without shortness of breath
4) Alteration in nutritional intake due to nausea and vomiting, labored		No c/o nausea / No vomiting / Taking liquids as offered	Eating solids / Takes in 50% each meal	Taking 50% each meal	Taking 50% each meal / Weight 2 lbs from patient's normal baseline	Taking 75% each meal	Taking 75% each meal
5) Potential for arrhythmias due to decreased cardiac output: decreased irritable foci, valve problems, decreased gas exchange	No evidence of life-threatening dysrhythmias	Normal sinus rhythm with benign ectopy	K(WNL) / Benign or no arrhythmias	Digoxin level WNL / Benign or no arrhythmias	Digoxin level WNL / Benign or no arrhythmias	Digoxin level WNL / Benign or no arrhythmias	Digoxin level WNL / Benign or no arrhythmias
6) Patient/family response to future treatment & hospitalization	Patient/family expressing concerns / Following directions of staff	Patient/family expressing concerns / Following directions of staff	Patient/family expressing concerns / Following directions of staff	States reasons for and cooperates with rest periods / Patient begins to assess own knowledge and ability to care for CHF at home	Patient decides whether he/she wants discussion with physician about advanced directives	States plan for 1–2 days postdischarge as to meds., diet, activity, follow-up appointments / Expresses reaction to having CHF	Repeats plans / States signs and symptoms to notify physician/ER / Signs discharge consent

TABLE 4-6 CAREMAP™: CONGESTIVE HEART FAILURE (*Continued*)

	Day 1	Day 1	Day 2	Day 3	Day 4	Day 5	Day 6
			Benchmark Quality Criteria				
Location	ER 1–4 hours	*Floor Telemetry or CCU 6–24 hours*	*Floor*	*Floor*	*Floor*	*Floor*	*Floor*
7) Individual problem:							
Staff Tasks							
			Critical Path (Interventions)				
Assessments/Consults	Vital signs q 15 min Nursing assessments focus on lung sounds, edema, color, skin integrity, jugular vein distention Cardiac monitor Arterial line if needed Swan-Ganz Intake & output	Vital signs q 15 min–1 hr Repeat nursing assessments Cardiac monitor Arterial line Swan-Ganz Daily weight Intake & output	Vital signs q 4 hrs Repeat nursing assessments D/C cardiac monitor 24 hr D/C arterial and Swan-Ganz Daily weight Intake & output	Vital signs q 6 hrs Repeat nursing assessments Daily weight Intake & output	Vital signs q 6 hrs Repeat nursing assessments Daily weight Intake & output Nutrition consult	Vital signs q 6 hrs Repeat nursing assessments Daily weight Intake & output	Vital signs q 6 hrs Repeat nursing assessments Daily weight Intake & output
Specimens/Tests	Consider TSH studies Chest X-ray EKG CPK q 8 hr × 3 ABG if pulse Ox: (range)	B/G	Evaluate for ECHO			Chest X-ray Lytes, BUN, Creatinine	

	Lytes, Na, K, Cl, CO_2, Glucose, BUN, Creatinine, Digoxin (range)					
Treatments	O_2 or intubate IV or Heparin lock	O_2 IV or Heparin lock	IV or Heparin lock	DC pulse Ox if stable D/C IV or Heparin lock		
Medications	Evaluate for Digoxin Nitrodrip or paste Diuretics IV Evaluate for antiemetics Evaluate for antiarrhythmics	Evaluate for Digoxin Nitrodrip or paste Diuretics IV Evaluate for pre-load/after-load reducers K supplements Stool softeners	D/C Nitrodrip or paste Diuretics IV or PO K supplements Stool softeners Evaluate for nicotine patch	Change to PO Digoxin PO diuretics K supplements Stool softeners Nicotine patch if consent	PO diuretics K supplement Stool softeners Nicotine patch if consent	PO diuretics K supplement Stool softeners Nicotine patch if consent
Nutrition	None	Clear liquids	Cardiac, low-salt diet	Cardiac, low-salt diet	Cardiac, low-salt diet	Cardiac, low salt-diet
Safety/Activity	Commode Bedrest with head elevated Reposition patient q 2 hrs Bedrails up Call light available	Commode Bedrest with head elevated Dangle Reposition patient q 2 hrs Enforce rest periods Bedrails up Call light available	Commode Enforce rest periods Chair with assist ½ hr with feet elevated Bedrails up Call light available	Bathroom privileges Chair × 3 Bedrails up Call light available	Ambulate in hall × 2 Up ad lib between rest periods Bedrails up Call light available	Encourage ADLs that approximate activities at home Bedrails up Call light available

TABLE 4-6 CAREMAP™: CONGESTIVE HEART FAILURE (Continued)

	Day 1	Day 1	Day 2	Day 3	Day 4	Day 5	Day 6
				Benchmark Quality Criteria			
Location	ER 1-4 hours	Floor Telemetry or CCU 6-24 hours	Floor	Floor	Floor	Floor	Floor
Teaching	Explain procedures Teach chest pain scale and importance of reporting	Explain course, need for energy conservation Orient to unit and routine	Clarify CHF Dx and future teaching needs Orient to unit and routine Schedule rest periods Begin medication teaching	Importance of weighing self every day Provide smoking cessation information Review energy conservation schedule	Cardiac rehab level as indicated by consult Provide smoking cessation support Dietary teaching	Review CHF education material with patient	Reinforce CHF teaching
Transfer/Discharge Coordination	Assess home situation: notify significant other If no arrhythmias or chest pain, transfer to floor Otherwise transfer to ICU	Screen for discharge needs Transfer to floor	Consider Home Health Care referral		Evaluate needs for diet and anti-smoking classes Physician offers discussion opportunities for advanced directives	Appointment and arrangement for follow-up care with Home Health Care nurses Contact VNA	Reinforce follow-up appointments

Reproduced by permission. CareMap® is a registered trademark and intellectual property of the Center for Case Management, South Natick, MA.

108

restoration of normal functioning and may take days to months to achieve. Intermediate outcomes describe client behavior in smaller steps. They might be more appropriate in a hospital where the client only stays a few days or in a more critical care setting when the client is unstable and the problem must be reduced or eliminated rapidly. Intermediate outcomes may be set in a time frame from hours to days. They are progressive and are used to show continued advancement, in terms of improved level of client functioning, in the direction of long-term or discharge outcome. An outcome statement contains the client behavior, the criteria of acceptable performance of that behavior, the time frame in which the outcome should be achieved, and the conditions, if any, under which the behavior will be demonstrated. Outcomes are realistic, observable, congruent with other health professional's plans of care, and directly related to the nursing diagnosis.

Nursing interventions are those specific activities the nurse plans and implements in order to help the client achieve an outcome. There are four broad categories of nursing interventions and the plan of care often incorporates actions from several of these groups: environmental management, physician-ordered and initiated interventions, physician-ordered/nurse-initiated interventions, and nurse-ordered/nurse-initiated interventions. The last group of interventions is solely within the realm of nursing practice and includes: health teaching, counseling, and referral; specific nursing treatments; medication administration; assisting with activities of daily living (ADL's); assessment of client status, progress, and response; assistance with problem solving; discharge planning; maximizing nutrition; and providing encouragement and hope. Nursing interventions deal with the problem and the etiology or risk factors identified in the nursing diagnosis and try to reduce or eliminate them. If that is not possible, interventions are aimed at lessening the problematic signs and symptoms to assist the client and family cope with the problem. Nursing interventions are safe for the client, specific, congruent with plans of other health care professionals and realistic for the client, the nurse, and the health care setting.

CASE STUDY: CARE PLAN (OUTCOMES, INTERVENTIONS, AND RATIONALE)

The care plan for Mrs. Witten follows. The data base and nursing diagnoses were developed in Chapters 2 and 3. A standard care plan form is also shown to illustrate how the nursing diagnosis of pain might be individualized.

CARE PLAN FOR MRS. WITTEN

Nursing Diagnoses	Outcomes	Interventions	Rationale
Pain secondary to possible cholecystitis	Report of pain at level of 4 or less during hospitalization	1. assess and elim. contributing factors 2. enc. alt. pain mgmt techniques 3. assess q3h; prn analgesic 4. reposition q2h	○ to lessen or elim. cause of pain ○ block or lessen pain perception ○ provide adequate drug level ○ reduce muscle strain ○ good body alignment increases comfort
Fear r/t illness, possible surgery or laparoscopic cholecystectomy	Client verbalizes decreased fear prior to tests, tx, surgery	1. manage pain 2. orient to room, routines 3. assess knowledge of illness, txs, info. from MD 4. explanations; clarify prior to all nsg/medical tests, tx 5. enc. family support 6. assess for concerns; need to talk 7. assess status q1–2h × 12h	○ pain can increase fear ○ decrease fear of unknown ○ begin to teach at level of understanding; fear can decrease perception/ understanding ○ decreases fear of unknown ○ presence of family can decrease fear/ anxiety ○ verbalizing fears can lessen them and allows nurse to correct misinformation ○ meets safety need

Nursing Diagnoses	Outcomes	Interventions	Rationale
Alt. health maintenance r/t knowledge deficit on BSE	Client to demo. BSE before disch.	1. explain impt. of early detection and tx	○ motivational
		2. discuss timing of BSE q mo 1–2 days post-menstruation	○ for consistency
		3. teach BSE techniques; normal and abnormal findings	○ for accurate dx of BSE findings
		4. demo/return demo of BSE	○ to assess learning
		5. BSE pamphlet	○ for home reference

Developed by: *L. Atkinson*
date: *6/3/94*

89714530
Witten, Laura
6/3/94 room 511
Dr. Ronal/Keller
Addressograph

NURSING DIAGNOSIS STANDARD CARE PLAN: PAIN

Pain related to *possible cholecystitis 6/3*
_____

("A state in which an individual experiences and reports the presence of
severe discomfort or an uncomfortable sensation," NANDA, 1992)
Client Characteristics: *reports RUQ pain, restless, P96, R28, BP 138/88*

Client Goals/Outcome Standards:
✓ Verbalization that pain has been eliminated or decreased to a level of
____4____ on a scale of 1–10 by *1 hr &*.
                    during *hospitalization*_____.
___ Evaluation: _____
✓ Reduction in values of vital signs: P, R, BP, toward normal range
    by __*1 hr*__.
___ Evaluation: _____
Other: _____
___ Evaluation: _____

Nursing Intervention Standards:
1. Assess pain and related factors.
   a. intensity (1–10) _rated as 8 on admission_
   b. duration _continuous; previously lasted several hours_
   c. character (sharp, dull, shooting, burning) _"acute" sharp_
   d. location _Right Upper quadrant_
   e. precipitated by _unknown_
2. Assess for effectiveness of previous pain relief interventions
   a. previous medication (drug, dose, route, effectiveness on 1–10) _____
      ASA 10 gr taken at home "not helpful at all, made me nauseated"
   b. other helpful measures: _____

3. Offer _Demerol 50-100 mg IM_ (analgesic ordered by MD) q _3-4 h_ prn.
4. Encourage use of analgesics before _tests_
   (pain precipitating activity) at _____ am/pm or _____
5. Offer relaxation techniques: slow relaxed breathing _explained 6/3_
                         music _____
                         backrub _qhs_
                         heat _____

6. Assist with repositioning as needed q _4° position of comfort_
7. Encourage use of distracting stimuli: radio, (TV), other: _____
   effleurage/skin stroking _RUQ by patient ad lib_

Developed by _L. Atkinson R.N._   date: _6/3/94_
Evaluated by _____ date: _____
Reviewed/Updated by _____ date: _____

Implementation

Like the other steps comprising the nursing process, the implementation phase consists of several activities: validating the care plan, writing the care plan, giving and documenting nursing care, and continuing to collect data.

$$\text{Implementing} = \frac{\text{Validating}}{\text{Care Plan}} + \frac{\text{Documenting}}{\text{Care Plan}} + \frac{\text{Giving and}}{\text{Documenting}} + \frac{\text{Continuing}}{\text{Data}}$$
Nursing Care   Collection

VALIDATING THE CARE PLAN

When nursing students or inexperienced staff nurses write care plans, it is recommended that they take the proposed care plans to a colleague and request validation. This step does not have to involve a lengthy scheduled consultation but is, rather, a very brief time during which nurses seek the opinion of other nurses. It is important that the student seek appropriate sources for validation. For example, the student may request the clinical instructor or responsible staff nurse to review the care plan. Such qualified sources can evaluate the care plan by using the following questions as guides.

1. Does the plan assure the client's safety?
2. Is the plan based on sound scientific principles?
3. Is the plan supported by accepted nursing knowledge?
4. Are the nursing diagnoses supported by the data? Are the major defining characteristics present?
5. Do priorities consider client preferences, physical and psychosocial needs?
6. Do the outcomes relate to the problems identified in the nursing diagnoses?
7. Do the outcomes contain a time and client behavior for evaluation?
8. Can the planned nursing actions realistically help the client to achieve the intended outcomes?
9. Are the nursing actions arranged in a logical sequence?
10. Is the plan individualized to the needs and capabilities of this particular client?
11. Is the plan congruent with the standards, protocols, and procedures for the particular health care setting? With plans of other health care professionals?

Thus, the nurse who provides the validation is reviewing the plan in four major areas:

1. Safety
2. Appropriateness
3. Effectiveness
4. Individualized nursing care

Because of their expertise in nursing care, other nurses are the most frequently used resource for validating. At times, a nurse may wish to utilize another health team member to review some aspect of a nursing care plan. For example, the nurse teaching a diabetic client about a diabetic exchange diet may wish to have a dietitian validate food substitutions requested by the client and family.

Occasionally, a nursing student may select an inappropriate person to validate a care plan. Frequently, nursing assistants are very knowledgeable about a specific type of care, having had several years' experience in a particular clinical area. However, the nursing student should not ask nursing assistants to validate a care plan. Nursing assistants may be a source for data in that they may be able to provide information about routines of the clinical area, but they are not planners of nursing care. This is a function of the professional nurse.

Having reviewed the plan with another nursing professional, the student or nurse may wish to share the completed plan with the client, who is another possible source for validation. The client or family can advise the nurse if any aspect of the plan is unacceptable. This gives clients another opportunity to participate in planning their own care. In summary, to validate the plan is to request another appropriate professional and the client, if possible, to give the plan approval for implementation.

DOCUMENTING THE NURSING CARE PLAN

To retain a nursing care plan for the exclusive use of one nurse is to defeat a primary purpose of care plans. In order to get the maximum effect, a care plan must get the maximum press!

A nurse may plan a client care conference as a "press conference" for a completed care plan. At such a meeting the nurse summarizes data, problems, outcomes, and planned actions. The nurse spends most of the time focusing on presenting the care plan to other nurses. At such a time the nurse may also gain new information to add to the care plan. This conference may be used as a problem-solving session during which a nurse may request assistance from colleagues to further develop a care plan.

Interdisciplinary care conferences involve various professionals such as the physician, physical therapist, social worker, dietician, and chaplain in addition to the client's primary nurse. All these professionals work together to develop a plan of care for the client, especially focusing on long-term outcomes and interventions. The client and family participate in this problem-solving group whenever possible.

The change of shift report is another time when the nurse shares concerns about clients, seeks additional data or suggestions from colleagues, identifies problems, sets priorities, identifies intermediate outcomes, and plans interventions. This process will direct the nurse's activities during the coming 8-hour shift. The nurse can delegate or clarify activities for other health team members so everyone knows what is important to assess and report and what to do for or with the client/family over the next few hours.

Another communication tool following the sequence of activities in the nursing process is a charting format known as a problem-oriented medical record (POMR). The plan of care in such a system then takes the form of SOAP or (SOAPIER) notes. The word SOAP is used as an acronym for *s*ubjective data, *o*bjective data, *a*ssessment, and *p*lan. Some formats add the use of the letters IER to include *i*mplementation, *e*valuation, and *r*eassessment.

Another popular format is "focus charting." The focus is often the diagnostic category or an identified nursing diagnosis. The charting then involves continued reporting of data on the problem, an interpretation of that data in relationship to the problem, changes or additions to nursing actions, and evaluation of outcomes after implementing these interventions.

Other hospitals use a nursing Kardex as a system of organizing care plans.

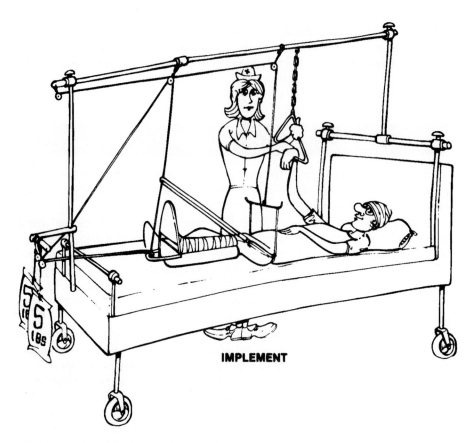

IMPLEMENT

FIGURE 5-1.   The real focus of a well-developed plan—giving the client quality nursing care.

A nursing Kardex is a file that contains the nursing care plans. Each plan is recorded on an oversized index card or large folded sheet of paper. Kardex forms may include space for medical treatments, diagnostic procedures, and other schedules. Still other institutions have adopted 8 1/2 inch × 11 inch nursing care plan forms, which have the advantage of corresponding to standard chart size.

Some hospitals are using the computer to generate a standardized care plan for a client with a specific diagnosis. The nurse begins with this care plan and then modifies it to meet the needs of the individual client. Other health care settings are "filling in the blanks" to individualize a preprinted standard care plan developed by more expert nurses.

The form of the written care plan may vary from institution to institution, but it should be a useful tool for communicating. Most will include space for nursing diagnoses, outcomes, nursing interventions, and evaluation in an abbreviated form. A written care plan may be condensed but must convey all essential information. Often nurses will use worksheets to record those problems, intermediate outcomes, and interventions that will probably be accomplished during their 8-hour shift.

This 8-hour plan does not need to be written as a permanent care plan, although the nursing care must be documented in the client's chart and a report given to the following shift of nurses. The written care plan should be used to communicate outcomes achieved by the client.

The following suggestions will assist the nurse to write a care plan.

1. Abbreviate whenever possible, using standardized medical or English symbols.
2. Choose key words to communicate ideas; do not write whole sentences.
3. Refer people to procedure books rather than trying to include all the steps for a procedure on a written plan.
4. Category headings should include nursing diagnoses, outcomes, nursing actions, and outcome evaluations.
5. The nursing diagnosis with the related outcomes, and nursing actions, should appear on the care plan.
6. Include a date for evaluation of each outcome.
7. All long-term outcomes should be written. Nursing actions directly related to long-term outcomes should also be written. If intermediate outcomes will be evaluated within the nurse's 8-hour shift, it is not necessary to include them on the written form. It is necessary to document the nursing care and the client outcome which actually occurred.
8. Intermediate outcomes that cannot be met within an 8-hour shift should be written in order that other nurses can continue the plan of care.
9. Long-term outcomes being met by a series of intermediate outcomes belong on the Kardex and/or in the client's chart. The accompanying actions for intermediate outcomes are included. If the intermediate outcome is to be met during the next few hours by the nurse writing the care plan, the nurse should write the next progressive intermediate outcome and nursing actions.
10. When intermediate outcomes are evaluated, they should be signed and dated by the responsible nurse.
11. All nursing interventions (actions, orders, or whatever term is being used) should be signed by the registered nurse responsible for writing them.

The nursing care plan for Mrs. Witten as it might appear on a Kardex or client's chart is at the end of this chapter.

GIVING AND DOCUMENTING NURSING CARE

At last! The nurse now has a plan that will individualize the care given to a client. Now the nurse is ready to give the care as planned. Even though the nurse has developed an excellent care plan, occasionally (and in the hospital it seems to be the rule), situations occur that interfere with implementing the plan. The client may be scheduled for emergency surgery. A client may be in great pain, which alters priorities. Visitors may arrive and the client is eager to spend time with them. In each case the nurse may be unable to implement the care plan without making some modifications. There are times when the nurse believes that performance of certain assessments, treatments, and activities are necessary for the client's physical safety. Clients, families, and other health care workers may then have to reset their priorities, reschedule, or modify what they were planning. For example, a newborn with an admitting rectal temperature of 96°F is hypothermic, and interventions to stabilize and raise the temperature should be implemented immediately. Any activities with the newborn, such as bathing or removing the baby from the warmer, might worsen the problem or interfere with treatment and should be delayed until the temperature is back in the normal range. The nurse discusses the problem, desired outcome, and interventions with the family and others working with

Even the best laid plans sometimes run amok . . .

. . . . I was a nursing instructor working with a young attractive, single male nursing student on the labor and delivery area. We had discussed how uncomfortable he felt and he jokingly said his goal for this clinical rotation was to avoid seeing a birth. We laughed, but I said I could accept that as long as he was responsible for the theoretical content and had some experience with the monitors and assessments. His eyes lit up as he scanned the Kardex and chose to follow two women in preterm labor where the goal of medical management was to stop their labor. When he began to follow them, both women were experiencing almost no contractions but had on fetal and uterine monitors. He was feeling quite smug with his assignment and relieved that it looked like his personal goal was a "given." As he walked past a patient's room on the way to the desk, he heard the patient scream out "Help! Help! The baby's coming!" He confided later that the thought crossed his mind to keep on walking but he stopped and went in. The woman was in a small panic and a look under the covers at the bulging perineum confirmed the reason for her distress. Just then the staff nurse the student was working with on the cases in preterm labor came into the room responding to the call light. "Saved!" he thought as he headed for the door. His nurse told him, in no uncertain terms, he was helping her and within a few minutes they had delivered the baby. I knew nothing of all this but I ran into him about 15 minutes after the birth and casually asked if he had gotten down for supper yet. "Supper!" he replied. "I just delivered a baby! I may never eat again!"

this newborn. The nurse may do some problem solving with the family at this time to identify alternate ways to meet family needs while still guaranteeing treatment for the hypothermia. For example, parents could keep the baby in their room under the warmer for picture taking and to prevent separation.

Finally, as a last step in implementation, the nurse documents the care given to clients, and their response. The nurse is guided by the old maxim "If it is not recorded, it has not been done." If evidence of implementation does not exist in the client's permanent record, it would seem that the plan has not been followed and the efforts of the nurse have been wasted. In addition, following the nursing interventions planned by a colleague is a way that nurses support each other in developing accountability for nursing care. Few nurses would omit giving or documenting a medication ordered by a physician. The implementation of nursing interventions is equally important to the well-being of clients and thus deserves to be treated seriously, respectfully, and with full accountability.

CONTINUING DATA COLLECTION

Throughout the process of implementation the nurse continues to collect data. As the client's condition changes, the data base changes, subsequently requiring revising and updating of the care plan. Data gathered while giving nursing care may also be used as evidence for evaluation of outcome achievement, which will be discussed in the next chapter.

IMPLEMENTATION: THE NEXT GENERATION

The first step in the implementation phase of the nursing process is validating the care plan. In the case management model, nurses and physicians have already validated the plan through the process of developing the tools of critical pathways, or CareMaps®. The tools represent these experts' ideas on what is the best care for a group of average clients admitted under the same DRG. It reflects a multidisciplinary approach with the actions of all involved health care professionals identified on a time grid. How a nurse actually works with the client and family to implement selected interventions in a plan of care changes with technology. But regardless of the health care delivery system, the nurse responds to the client's current status and needs when giving direct care. The nurse is directing interventions toward achieving *outcomes* in all delivery systems.

With case management, and the use of critical pathways or CareMaps,® the nurse's role in validating the plan as appropriate for this client and individualizing care is more crucial. This is because the care plan was not based

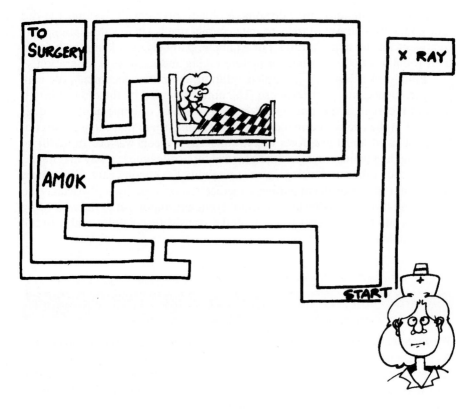

FIGURE 5-2. Even the best laid plans sometimes run amok.

on one individual's data base but on the common needs and problems of a large group of clients admitted under the same DRG. The suggestion is made that when using the CareMap® system, the nurse consider the following questions while implementing care:

1. What interventions and outcomes should be happening during this shift?
2. What is actually happening?
3. What did not happen, and why?
4. What should be done about it?
5. Who will rectify it, and when?

(Zander, in Melum et al., 1992, p. 310.)

SUMMARY

Implementation is the fourth step in the nursing process, and the focus is on the nurse working with the client to carry out the plan of care. Implementation consists of validating the care plan (is it a safe, reasonable plan indicating quality nursing care?), and documenting and communicating it, but the primary component is actually giving care to the client. The nurse then documents this care and the client's response to it in the chart. As the nurse gives care, assessment of the client continues. This is done not only to see how the client responds to the nursing interventions but to provide increased information for revising the plan of care as client status changes. The client is an active participant in care, working with the nurse to adapt interventions as they are given and having the right to refuse or request interventions. The nurse is flexible, open to suggestions and changing client and family priorities, but committed to helping them understand and accept nursing care to promote health and reduce, eliminate, or prevent problems.

CASE STUDY: ABBREVIATED CARE PLAN

ABBREVIATED CARE PLAN FOR MRS. WITTEN

Nursing Diagnoses	Outcomes	Interventions	Outcome Evaluation
Pain r/t possible cholecystitis	Report of pain at level of 4 or less during hospitalization	1. assess and elim. contributing factors 2. enc. alt. pain mgmt techniques 3. assess q3h; prn analgesic 4. reposition q2h	_____
Fear r/t illness, possible surgery, or laparoscopic cholecystectomy	Client verbalizes decreased fear prior to tests, tx, surgery	1. manage pain 2. orient to room, routines 3. assess knowledge of illness, txs, info. from MD 4. explanations; clarify prior to all nsg/medical tests, tx 5. enc. family support 6. assess for concerns; need to talk 7. assess status q1–2h × 12h	_____

Nursing Diagnoses	Outcomes	Interventions	Outcome Evaluation
Alt. health maintenance r/t knowledge deficit on BSE	Client to demo. BSE before disch.	1. explain impt. of early detection and tx 2. discuss timing of BSE q mo 1–2 days post menstruation 3. teach BSE techniques; normal and abnormal findings 4. demo./return demo. of BSE 5. BSE pamphlet	_____

Developed by: *L. Atkinson, RN*   date: *6/3/94*

Evaluation

Evaluation occurs continuously while giving care, shift by shift, as nurses evaluate progress toward intermediate outcomes; and summatively at discharge from the health care facility with the evaluation of discharge outcomes. There are four distinct activities in the evaluation phase of the nursing process.

Evaluating =	Documenting Responses to Interventions	+	Evaluating Effectiveness of Interventions	+	Evaluating Outcome Achievement	+	Reviewing Nursing Care Plan

DOCUMENTING RESPONSES TO INTERVENTIONS

While giving care to the client, the nurse continually evaluates how the client is responding to the interventions. The client may be responding in the way the nurse expected—the way most clients respond. In this situation the nursing treatment or action produced the expected result, and the nurse will describe this response in the client's chart or on whatever form of documentation the health care facility is using. "Client tolerated standing at bedside and walking to bathroom with only minor dizziness on first ambulation postoperatively."

Perhaps the client may have responded in an unexpected way, either positively or negatively. The nurse documents this response too, but usually has to adapt the subsequent interventions planned because of this unexpected response. The alteration in subsequent interventions is then documented along with the client's response. "Client became very dizzy and slightly nauseated when standing at bedside while attempting first ambulation postop. Patient returned to bed. Instructed not to attempt getting out of bed without assistance." Now the nurse has to select new nursing interventions on the spot, based on these client reactions to the attempted ambulation. The nurse assesses the vital signs, gives the client a cool washcloth for the face, reassures the client that this response is not unusual and that the next attempt will go better. The nurse shares the modified plan to delay ambulating again until the client has had a chance to take in some food and fluids over the next few hours. For the client's safety, the nurse emphasizes that the client should not attempt to get out of bed without a nurse to help. This is an example of the kind of ongoing evaluation of the client and adaptation of the planned interventions that goes on continuously while giving care. All aspects of this process are documented: the action(s), the client response(s) and the adaptations made in the interventions, and later the client response following the adapted interventions.

EVALUATING EFFECTIVENESS OF INTERVENTIONS

The nurse using the nursing process is always aware of the intermediate and discharge outcomes selected as goals for client behaviors following nursing interventions. Interventions are evaluated in terms of their usefulness in assisting the client to move toward these outcomes. Nursing interventions are selected based on scientific principles and nursing knowledge. They are supposed to produce a specific result when used with most clients. If the nursing interventions produce the expected result in client behavior, they are effective and will advance the client toward the outcome. If the interventions produce an unexpected result or are not possible to implement at the expected time because of variations in an individual's response or speed of recovery, the interventions need to be examined to try to improve their effectiveness. Questions the nurse can ask as interventions are evaluated include:

1. Was there a language barrier or cultural orientation of the nurse or the client that reduced the effectiveness of the intervention? What can be done to remedy this?

2. Do I need more skill or practice to make this intervention more effective?
3. Did I consider approaching the problem from many different angles, or did I use only one intervention? (For example, giving an analgesic when requested by the client, versus exploration of the pain to try to eliminate precipitating factors combined with other pain management strategies in addition to medication.)
4. Would my interventions be more effective if the family or significant others were more involved? less involved?
5. Did I share the plan with the client to promote understanding and participation?
6. Do I need to seek out the expertise of another nurse to suggest interventions, adaptations of interventions, or resequencing of interventions that would be more effective?
7. Did the client's condition change, making the type and timing of the interventions less appropriate and therefore less effective?

EVALUATION OF OUTCOME ACHIEVEMENT

The purpose of this part of the evaluation is to decide whether the client has achieved the outcomes selected during the planning phase of the nursing process. The outcomes are evaluated at the time or date specified in the plan. While giving care, the nurse is continuously collecting new data about the client. Some of this information will be used for evaluation of outcome achievement. When evaluating outcome achievement, the nurse returns to the outcome statement in the care plan. What was the specific client behavior stated in the desired outcome? Was the client able to perform the behavior by the time allowed in the outcome statement? Was the client able to perform the behavior as well as described in the criteria part of the outcome statement? The answers to these questions are the basis for an evaluation of outcome achievement.

The only thing that is evaluated is the client's ability to demonstrate the behavior described in the outcome statement. Nursing actions are not evaluated at this point and are not part of the evaluation statement. Effectiveness of the nursing actions and teaching plans will be examined separately. The nurse may have given the world's fastest bedbath, but that is not important for evaluating outcome achievement. If the intermediate outcome was to have the client relax and sleep for several hours, the nurse evaluates the client's behavior. Did the client sleep for several hours? The skill with which a nurse performs various procedures is important and will affect outcome achievement. However, when an evaluative statement is written, it is the client's behavior or condition that is assessed. *The result of nursing care in the form of changed client behavior or condition is the focus of outcome-based evaluation.*

Writing an Evaluative Statement

There are two parts to an evaluative statement: a decision on how well the outcome was achieved, and the client data or behavior that supports this decision. The nurse has three alternatives when deciding how well an outcome was met: (1) met, (2) partially met, and (3) not met.

If the client was able to demonstrate the behavior by the specific time or date in the outcome statement, the outcome was met. If the client was able to demonstrate the behavior but not as well as the nurse had specified in the outcome statement, the outcome was partially met. If the client was unable or unwilling to perform the behavior at all, the outcome was not met.

$$
\begin{array}{c}
\text{Outcome} \\
\text{Evaluation Statement}
\end{array}
=
\begin{array}{c}
\text{Outcome Met} \\
\text{Outcome Partially} \\
\text{Met Outcome} \\
\text{Not Met}
\end{array}
+
\begin{array}{c}
\text{Actual Client} \\
\text{Behavior} \\
\text{as Evidence}
\end{array}
$$

In the second part of the evaluation statement, the nurse includes a description of the client's actual behavior as the individual tries to demonstrate the behavior identified in the outcome. For example, if the behavior identified in the outcome was for the client to report some degree of pain relief, the nurse talks with the client regarding severity of pain, following the nursing interventions to help relieve it. The client's response about the severity of current pain makes up the second part of the outcome evaluative statement. Another example might be:

1. Nursing Diagnosis: Activity intolerance related to prolonged bedrest.
   Outcome Statement: Client will walk length of hall and back by 2/7.
   Outcome Evaluation (done on 2/7 or earlier):
   Outcome achieved; client walked length of hall and back.
   Outcome partially achieved; client walked length of hall but too tired to walk back.
   Outcome not achieved; client refused to walk.
   Outcome not achieved; client unable to bear his own weight.
2. Nursing Diagnosis: Impaired tissue integrity related to pressure and poor circulation.
   Outcome Statement: 2/7 Decubitus ulcer (bedsore) will be healed in 1 month.
   Outcome Evaluation (done on 3/7 or earlier):
   Outcome met; decubitus ulcer healed.
   Outcome partially met; decubitus ulcer still present but is 1/2 the size and dry.
   Outcome not met; decubitus ulcer broken open and draining.

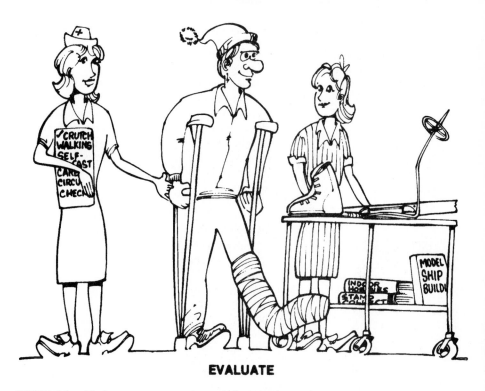

EVALUATE

FIGURE 6-1.   Discharge outcome achieved. Congratulations!

3. Nursing Diagnosis: Noncompliance with assigned reading in *Understanding the Nursing Process* related to belief content is "boring."
    Outcome Statement: After finishing Chapter 6, the student will state this nursing process book is the most interesting book ever read.
    Outcome Evaluation (done when the student finishes Chapter 6):
    Outcome met; student stated this book was the most interesting book ever read and asked for an "A" in the course.
    Outcome partially met; student said this book was about as interesting as any other course books, and asked for a "C" in the course.
    Outcome not met: student lost book and asked for a class withdrawal slip.

Client Participation and Evaluation

Evaluation of outcome achievement is done with the client whenever possible. It may also be done with the client's family. It is not just the nurse's assessment of the client's ability to achieve an outcome that is important. The client's perception is also important since the problem identified in the nursing diagnosis is the client's problem and not the nurse's. The client who evaluates personal outcome achievement is a partner with the nurse and receives feed-

TABLE 6–1   EVALUATION OF OUTCOMES

Nursing Diagnoses	Outcomes	Outcome Evaluation
1. Knowledge deficit of diabetic management related to new diagnosis	1. Maintains control of blood glucose levels from 80–180 m/dl (long-term outcome) a. accurately checks blood glucose level QID before discharge (intermediate outcome) b. lists signs and symptoms of hyperglycemia and hypoglycemia by 11/12 (intermediate outcome) c. states actions to take for hyper/hypoglycemia by 11/12 (intermediate outcome) d. correctly administers own insulin by discharge (intermediate outcome or discharge outcome) e. correctly explains how to adjust diet and insulin with short-term illness by 11/13 (intermediate outcome)	a. outcome met; correctly performed self blood glucose checks × 4 *L. Atkinson R.N. 11/11/94* b. outcome partially met; lists S&S for hypoglycemia, confused on hyperglycemia *L. Atkinson R.N. 11/12/94* c. outcome met; stated corrective actions for hyper/hypoglycemia *L. Atkinson R.N. 11/12/94* d. outcome met; correctly gave self mixed dose of NPH and Regular insulin × 2 days *L. Atkinson R.N. 11/14/94* e. outcome not met; states never sick and does not think adjustment necessary *L. Atkinson R.N. 11/13/94*
2. Fear related to development of diabetes and complications which may develop	2. Client to state decreased fear and confidence in ability to reduce risks of complications by 11/14 (long-term outcome)	2. Outcome met. States "it will be a constant worry but I am not as terrified as I was. Lots of people do fine managing their diabetes." *L. Atkinson R.N. 12/14/94*
3. Body image disturbance related to diagnosis of insulin dependent diab. as evidenced by anger over need to take insulin and change lifestyle	3. Verbalizations of acceptance of diab. and willingness to make changes by 12/14 (long-term outcome)	3. Outcome not met; client states anger about dx and states it's not fair. "I just hate taking shots; it makes me feel like a drug addict" *L. Atkinson R.N. 12/14/94*

back on progress toward eliminating or reducing the original problem identified in the nursing diagnosis. When a client successfully achieves an outcome mutually set with the nurse, that person receives positive reinforcement to continue efforts toward a higher level of functioning.

When evaluating outcome achievement, the nurse is responsible for documenting both parts of the outcome statement. The nurse doing the evaluation with the client includes the date the evaluation was done, whether or not the outcome was achieved, subjective and objective data related to the client's behavior compared to the behavior identified in the outcome, and the nurse's signature. This information is all recorded on the chart or care plan. See Table 6-1. The care plan for Mrs. Witten, developed in Chapters 2, 3, 4, and 5 is presented in Table 6-2 with the addition of evaluation of outcome achievement.

CASE STUDY: OUTCOME EVALUATION

REVIEW OF THE NURSING CARE PLAN

Following evaluation of outcome achievement, the nurse repeats the activities in the nursing process by reviewing the plan of care. This is done whether the outcome was achieved or not. Review of the nursing care plan keeps the plan current and responsive to the client's changing needs. The process of nursing is not just sequential, consisting of steps 1 through 5 and then you are done. The process of nursing is cyclical in nature, with the steps of assessment, diagnosis, planning, implementation, and evaluation viewed as a circle with one step leading to another. The nursing care a person receives reflects the changing health status of the client, medical treatment changes, environmental changes, and the changing needs of the client and family.

$$\text{Review of the Nursing Care Plan} = \text{Reassessment} + \text{Review of Nursing Diagnoses} + \text{Replanning} + \text{Review of Implementation}$$

Review of the care plan using the nursing process consists of activities already described in the previous chapters: reassessment, review of diagnoses, replanning, and review of implementation. This process of review results in an updated plan for nursing care, which is then implemented and evaluated, leading again to review as part of evaluation.

TABLE 6–2   ABBREVIATED CARE PLAN FOR MRS. WITTEN (EVALUATION ADDED)

Nursing Diagnoses	Outcomes	Interventions	Evaluation Outcome
Pain secondary to possible cholecystitis	Report of pain at level of 4 or less during hospitalization	1. assess and elim. contributing factors 2. enc. alt. pain mgmt techniques 3. assess q3h; prn analgesic 4. reposition q2h	Partially met; client reported pain tolerable with analgesic but still hurts, 6/6/94 *L. Atkinson R.N.*
Fear r/t illness, possible surgery	Client verbalizes decreased fear prior to tests, tx, surgery	1. manage pain 2. orient to room, routines 3. assess knowledge of illness, txs, info. from MD 4. explanations; clarify prior to all nsg/medical tests, tx 5. enc. family support 6. assess for concerns; need to talk 7. assess status q1-2h × 12h	Partly met; reporting "scared" but better than at admission. 6/5/94 *L. Atkinson R.N.*
Alt. health maintenance r/t knowledge deficit on BSE	Client to demo. BSE before disch.	1. explain impt of early detection & tx 2. discuss timing of BSE q mo 1–2 days post menstruation 3. teach BSE techniques; normal & abnormal findings 4. demo/return demo of BSE 5. BSE pamphlet	Met; client demo. BSE correctly 6/8/94 *M. Burns R.N.*

Developed by: *L. Atkinson R.N.*   date: *6/3/94*

Reassessment

The process of reassessment results in an updated information base on the client. The nurse is continually assessing the client during all interactions. This accumulation of new data will now supplement the original data base from which the care plan was developed. After evaluation of intermediate outcome achievement, the nurse looks at the data, the diagnosis, desired outcomes and interventions again. In reassessment, the nurse:

1. Examines original data (related to the problem and intermediate outcome just evaluated) to decide whether it still accurately represents the client's status.
2. Examines new data gathered during interventions with the client to: clarify the original problem, its etiology, and related signs and symptoms; serve as a data base for a new nursing diagnosis.

Review of Nursing Diagnoses

The end product of reviewing the nursing diagnoses is a care plan containing only those diagnoses that are current or high-risk problems for the client. This may result in the same diagnoses continuing as part of the plan, new diagnoses being added, and resolved diagnoses eliminated. During the process of reviewing diagnoses, the nurse:

1. Analyzes new data to determine if a new problem exists and makes a new nursing diagnosis as needed. This addition is then documented in the care plan.
2. Analyzes original and new data including data from outcome evaluation to determine if original diagnoses are still accurate, current problems requiring nursing care. If they are still accurate and current, these diagnoses remain on the care plan as originally written.
3. Clarifies diagnostic statements to reflect any changes or additions in etiology or signs and symptoms discovered during ongoing assessment with the client. These changes are then added to the original diagnostic statement in the chart.
4. Analyzes original and new data, and data from outcome evaluation to determine if the problem has been resolved and no longer requires nursing care. "Diagnosis resolved" is then documented and dated on the chart, and nurses no longer perform the interventions associated with that diagnosis.

If the outcome was not achieved, reassessment and review of the diagnoses may help to point out reasons for this, such as inaccurate or incomplete data, inaccurate analysis of the data resulting in an invalid nursing diagnosis, or the development of new problems that interfered with the original plan. If the outcome was met and the problem resolved, the nurse considers the need for preventive nursing care if the client is still at risk.

A student in nursing discovers the problem when review of the care plan is not complete . . .

. . . *I was teaching with a group of 3rd quarter nursing students on an orthopedic clinical area. We had spent a lot of classroom and clinical time on developing nursing care plans, but in the actual clinical setting the students found standard care plans being used. Nurses would diagnose a problem area based on patient assessment and then use the NANDA-approved diagnoses with suggested goals and interventions all typed out. The nurse was to individualize this care plan based on knowledge of the patient and the medical treatment plan and put it in the chart. Well, the students were thrilled. This was a lot better than creating a care plan from scratch. A few words and marks on a preprinted form and they were done. One student in particular was irritated with the nursing faculty for making the students do all this work of care planning when in reality the nurses in the hospital were using care plan forms developed by experienced nurses from the health care facility. The Kardex only contained a list of partially written diagnoses such as "Pain" or "Impaired Physical Mobility." I expressed my concern that care plan review could easily be neglected by such a process because many nurses do not use the chart as a guide to nursing care but continue to use the Kardex which no longer contains the plan of care. My fears were dismissed as unrealistic because on the flow sheet in the patient's chart each shift documented, by initialing, that the care plan had been reviewed. About an hour later, that student called me over and said she had a real problem. The patient she had been caring for all shift was a four day postop amputee. The student had found the plan of care and knew she had to read it because I would be around asking if it was updated. The diagnosis of "Pain related to poor circulation and skin breakdown areas on left lower leg" was still in the chart as originally individualized by the admitting nurse over a week ago. That lower leg had been amputated four days ago. "How could this happen?" she asked. I just smiled. The students had a great postconference discussion on charting, care planning, legal documentation, and ethics.*

Replanning

The outcome of this activity will be a plan of care ready for implementation based on current problems, with outcomes and interventions adjusted to best reflect the client's abilities and preferences. Ineffective interventions can be eliminated, effective ones emphasized, and new approaches included to facilitate movement toward achievement of discharge outcomes. During this step, the nurse:

1. Reexamines priorities among the diagnoses and determines if they are still appropriate. Priorities are reordered as needed based on new data, new diagnoses, medical management, and expected date for discharge, transfer, surgery, and so on.

2. Examines previous outcomes and determines if they are still appropriate or if the client's status has changed, making the outcomes unrealistic. The behavior, time frame, criteria, and condition can all be altered to make the intermediate outcomes and discharge outcomes more appropriate and achievable, while still moving toward problem resolution.

3. Identifies new outcomes for new diagnoses and selects interventions. These then are documented in the chart.

4. Examines nursing interventions selected in the original plan and determines whether they should continue unchanged or whether a different approach would be more effective. Any changes, additions, or deletions are then documented in the chart as part of the updated care plan.

Without reassessment by a nurse the client's recovery may have been at risk . . .

. . . . *I hate to float to another area when our floor isn't busy. But float me they did. I usually worked on the burn unit and really felt competent working with the patients but they floated me to an oncology/chemotherapy unit. Different treatments, different problems, different things to assess, lots of drugs to look up. One of my patients was a man admitted to the hospital for workup of an unidentified blood disorder that had been causing him trouble for 15 years. The focus of care was on his hematologic problem, pain management, and possible narcotic addiction. On the Kardex it was noted that he had a partial thickness burn on the palm of his hand that had been treated in the emergency room. The last date on the treatment order for the burn was a week ago. I knew what a burn of that degree should look like if it was healing properly, but his hand didn't look the way it should. I assessed the hand and reviewed the ordered treatment based on my own knowledge of burn healing, complications, and available treatments. I discussed my concerns with the head nurse, who admitted being unfamiliar with burn therapy and complications. She notified the responsible physician, who then asked for a consult from one of the physicians on the burn unit. The doctor came down and reassessed the burn and the treatment and told me it was a good thing I had questioned the healing and treatment. He said I had probably saved the patient from an infection and possible sepsis by my assessment and action. I guess some days nurses are meant to float.*

The following example illustrates review of the plan of care. The reader should understand these steps are not written out as such in the plan as are diagnoses, outcomes, and interventions; but the plan of care is continually updated using whatever form of documentation the health care setting has implemented. Therefore the nurse will not find the headings of "reassessment," "review of diagnoses," "review of plan," or "review of implementation" as part of the care plan. These steps indicate the *process* the nurse goes through to reach the *product* of an effective, current plan of care.

Nursing Diagnoses	Outcome	Interventions	Outcome Evaluation
High risk for impaired tissue integrity r/t cast on left leg. 6/4/94	Tissue to remain intact, with normal sensation while hospitalized in cast	1. Assess CMS qh × 24 then q4h 2. Elevate leg in good alignment × 24h 3. Turn and reposition q2h until cast dry 4. Pad friction areas at knee and toes	Date: 6/6/94 Eval: Outcome met; tissue intact at discharge

Developed by: *L. Atkinson R.N. 6/4/94*

Signature:
of nurse evaluating
L. Atkinson R.N.

New Data	New Updated Outcome	New Interventions
1. 6/6 discharge to home in cast. 2. Skin intact at discharge. (Original Dx still appropriate)	Tissue to remain intact, with normal sensation while casted	1. Assess knowledge of S&S of inadeq circ., pressure, friction 2. Teach home care of cast 3. Enc. elevation when sitting at home/work

Developed by: *L. Atkinson R.N. 6/6/94*

Review of Implementation

During review of implementation, the nurse examines what actually happened with the client and family during nursing care. Factors such as the environment, the nurse's skills and knowledge, and the client and family's responses are considered. This is where the nurse evaluates personal behavior in relation to giving care. Does the nurse require further skills or information to be more effective? Did the nurse's personal feelings or cultural bias affect the quality of care delivered to the client? Were the interventions realistic in terms of time and resources? Were the interventions carried out by other nursing or health care personnel? If not, why not? Were the interventions too vague or misinterpreted? Review of what occurred during implementation of the original nursing plan of care may point out problems that can be corrected as the plan is updated. This is especially important when the intermediate outcome or discharge outcome was not achieved. Evaluation helps the nurse develop the skills of writing realistic and effective care plans for dealing with a client's problems.

EVALUATION: THE NEXT GENERATION

In a case management model using the CareMap® tool, the variance component is where evaluation occurs. "A CareMap® document without the variance component is a process without evaluation" (Zander, 1992). The variance component of the CareMap® system "shows us how and why clinicians and patients differ from the norm, as well as where an institution might improve on its services" (Zander, 1992). In the variance tool the nurse documents how and why the client deviated from the expected results. These deviations may be changes from the expected schedule, or unexpected responses to nursing interventions. Intermediate and discharge outcomes are evaluated as in the traditional or standardized care plan system. When evaluating outcomes and interventions from the CareMap®, its creator suggests these options for evaluation:

1. "Yes," this intermediate goal or outcome was either met as described or "No," it wasn't met as described,
2. "Yes," this staff intervention occurred or "No," it did not occur as described; and
3. If "No," then a variance is considered to be present.

(Zander, Fall 1992, p. 1)

When charting the variance, the nurse who recognizes it records a description of what actually happened in the client's chart along with the action(s) taken. Hospitals can keep track of variances occurring because of a client's status, clinician or nurse differences, hospital events that might have caused a variance, and community events causing variance. (For example, delay in hospital discharge because of problems with nursing home placement.) With this data, changes in the CareMap® can be made to improve the quality and effectiveness of the plan and decrease the length of hospital stay. This process of evaluating the CareMap® involves interdisciplinary staff caring for clients in a given DRG category.

SUMMARY

Evaluation involves four activities. Documenting client responses to interventions and evaluating the effectiveness of those interventions are the first two activities. Another part of evaluation involves evaluation of outcome achievement. To do this, the nurse returns to the outcome to review the behavior identified which would indicate a lessening or elimination of an actual client problem. Using the new data collected during implementation of the care plan, the nurse evaluates the client's ability to demonstrate the outcome behavior. A range of outcomes can be expected from complete ability to demonstrate the behavior as stated, to complete inability or unwillingness to demonstrate the behavior. This evaluation is documented in the chart with a description of the client's outcome behavior as evidence of the degree of achievement.

The last part of evaluation is to review the entire plan of care. This involves updating the data base, deciding if original diagnoses are still accurate, adding new diagnoses or identifying original ones as resolved, revising the outcomes and interventions based on more complete information on the client and the effectiveness of the original plan, and finally implementing the updated plan. This is again followed by evaluation and care plan review to reflect the dynamic state of the client. (See Figure 6-2).

CASE STUDY: REVIEW OF CARE PLAN

The care plan of Mrs. Witten follows with the addition of review of the plan of care. The updated abbreviated care plan demonstrates how it might appear on a nursing Kardex or in the chart. Outcome evaluation on a standard care plan form for the diagnostic category of "Pain" as it might be individualized for Mrs. Witten is also shown.

ABBREVIATED CARE PLAN FOR MRS. WITTEN (UPDATED POSTOP)

Revisions in the care plan are indicated with a * to make changes more obvious, but they would not appear this way on an actual plan of care.

**1. EVALUATION OF
INTERMEDIATE GOAL
ACHIEVEMENT:**   outcome met   outcome not met

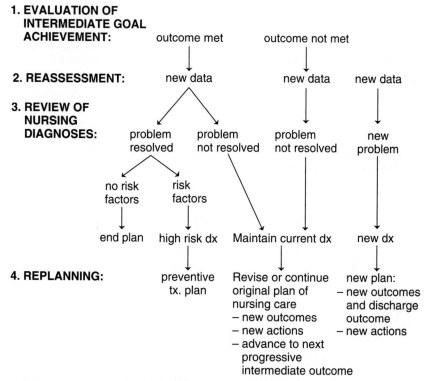

2. REASSESSMENT: new data   new data   new data

**3. REVIEW OF
NURSING
DIAGNOSES:**   problem   problem   problem   new
                    resolved   not resolved not resolved problem

                  no risk   risk
                  factors   factors

            end plan   high risk dx   Maintain current dx   new dx

4. REPLANNING: preventive   Revise or continue   new plan:
                            tx. plan   original plan of   – new outcomes
                                          nursing care   and discharge
                                          – new outcomes   outcome
                                          – new actions   – new actions
                                          – advance to next
                                            progressive
                                            intermediate outcome

5. REVIEW OF IMPLEMENTATION: How could the nurse do or schedule
things differently to be more effective? Improved skill or knowledge base
needed? Alter priorities? Better assessments? Help from other health care
professionals? Better delegation of responsibility to other nursing staff?

FIGURE 6-2.   Evaluation flow chart.

Reassessment: new data 6/6/94
—transferred back to station 3 hours postop, cholecystectomy
—IV infusing at 125cc/h, D5LR 1000cc to run × 3 liters
—Penrose drain in place draining blood-tinged bile
—½ inch diameter drainage area on incisional dressing
—nasogastric tube in place draining gastric contents on low suction
—NPO day of surgery, then clear liquids as tol. first postop day
—shallow respirations; 22–24 breaths/min
—reports severe incisional pain with movement, deep breathing
—refuses to cough; "hurts too much"
—moist breath sounds in lower left lung
—states, "I'm so glad it is over! What a relief"
—pulse 92, BP 142/70
—Demerol 50–100mg IM, prn pain
—Tylenol #3 1–2 tabs prn pain, first postop day

Nursing Diagnoses	Outcomes	Interventions	Outcome Evaluation
Pain secondary to possible cholecystitis 6/3/94	Report of pain at level of 4 or less during hospitalization	1. assess and elim. contributing factors 2. enc. alt. pain mgmt techniques 3. assess q3h prn analgesic 4. reposition q2h	Outcome partially met; pain reported tolerable with analgesics but still hurts. 6/4/94 *L. Atkinson R.N.*
*Pain related to surgery 6/3/94	*Report of pain at level of 4 or less with use of analgesics during hospitalization	*1. explain analgesia options: type and dose based on pain *2. enc. use of anal. before pain severe *3. pain assessment q 3–4h *4. assist with repositioning q2h *5. demo splinting incision for movement/ coughing/deep breath *6. call light in reach *7. backrub at hs	
Fear r/t illness, possible surgery 6/3/94	Client verbalizes decreased fear prior to tests, tx, surgery	1. manage pain as above 2. orient to room, routines 3. assess knowledge of illness txs, info. from MD 4. explanations; clarify prior to all nsg/medical tests, tx 5. enc. family support	Outcome partly met; reporting "scared" but better than at admission. 6/3/94 *L. Atkinson R.N.* Outcome met; problem resolved. Client expresses relief surgery over 6/3/94

Nursing Diagnoses	Outcomes	Interventions	Outcome Evaluation
		6. assess for concerns/need to talk	
		7. assess status ql–2h × 12h	
Alt. health maintenance r/t knowledge deficit on BSE 6/3/94	Client to demo. BSE before disch.	Schedule teaching for 6/4 1. explain impt of early detection and tx 2. discuss timing of BSE q mo 1–2 days post menstruation 3. teach BSE techniques; normal and abnormal findings 4. demo-return demo of BSE 5. BSE pamphlet	
*Ineffective airway clearance related to pain as evidenced by shallow resp. at 24, refusal to cough or deep breathe, moist breath sounds in L lower lung. 6/3/94	*Clear breath sounds by 6/4.	*1. explain need to cough deep breathe *2. assess breath sounds q4h *3. SMI × 3 qh (sustained maximal inspiration held for several seconds before exhale) *4. inspirometer q2h × 48h *5. reposition q2h *6. enc. use of analgesics, splinting to decrease pain so client will cough; enc. coughing	

Nursing Diagnoses	Outcomes	Interventions	Outcome Evaluation
		q2h until lungs clear	
		*7. begin ambulation 1st postop day and advance as tol.	
Developed by: *L. Atkinson R.N.*		date: *6/3/94*	
Reviewed/updated: *M. E. Murray R.N.*		date: *6/3/94*	

89714530
Witten, Laura
6/3/94, room 511
Dr. Ronal/Keller
Addressograph

NURSING DIAGNOSIS STANDARD CARE PLAN: PAIN

Pain related to *possible cholecystitis 6/3 0730*
6/6 1800 Pain related to laparoscopic surgery for cholecystitis
("A state in which an individual experiences and reports the presence of severe discomfort or an uncomfortable sensation," NANDA, 1992)
Client Characteristics: *reports RUQ pain, restless, P96, R28, BP 138/88*
6/6 Pt. reports post-op pain as 6, continuous dull, P90 R20, BP130/74
Client Goals/Outcome Standards:
✓ Verbalization that pain has been eliminated or decreased to a level of
____4____ on a scale of 1–10 by *1 hr &* .
during *hospitalization* .
6/3 Evaluation: *Outcome partly met; pt. reports pain tolerable c̄ analgesics but still hurts*
✓ Reduction in values of vital signs: P, R, BP, toward normal range
by *1 hr* .
6/3 Evaluation: *Outcome partially met; p88, R20, BP 130/76*
Other: *6/6 Pt. to state pain maintained at 4 or less during post-op recovery*
____ Evaluation: _____

Nursing Intervention Standards:
1. Assess pain and related factors.
    a. intensity (1–10) *rated as 8 on admission*
    b. duration *continuous; previously lasted several hours*
    c. character (sharp, dull, shooting, burning) *sharp*
    d. location *Right Upper quadrant*
    e. precipitated by *unknown*

2. Assess for effectiveness of previous pain relief interventions
   a. previous medication (drug, dose, route, effectiveness on 1–10) _____
      ASA 10 gr taken at home "not helpful at all, made me nauseated"
   b. other helpful measures: ══════════════════════════

3. Offer *Demerol 50-100 mg IM* (analgesic ordered by MD) q _3-4 h_ prn.
   6/6 Post-op Demerol 75-100 mg IM
4. Encourage use of analgesics before *tests* _____
   (pain precipitating activity) at _____ am/pm or _____
5. Offer relaxation techniques: slow relaxed breathing *explained 6/3*
                                 music ══════════════════════
                                 backrub *qhs* _____
                                 heat ══════════════════════
6. Assist with repositioning as needed q *4° position of comfort*
   6/6 Assist q 2° c̄ repositioning
7. Encourage use of distracting stimuli: radio, (TV), other: _____
   effleurage/skin stroking *RUQ by patient ad lib*
   6/6 Discourage effleurage

Developed by *L. Atkinson R.N.* _____ date: *6/3/94*
Evaluated by *L. Atkinson R.N.* _____ date: *6/3/94*
Reviewed/Updated by *L. Atkinson R.N.* _____ date: *6/6/94 1800*

Bibliography

AMERICAN NURSES ASSOCIATION (1991). *Standards of Clinical Nursing Practice.* Kansas City, MO, American Nurses Association, # NP.79.20M.

BENNER, P. (1984). *From Novice to Expert.* Menlo Park, CA, Addison-Wesley.

BOOTH, B., and WEBB, C. (February 12, 1992). One step forward or two steps back? *Nursing Times* 88(7):32–34.

BRIDER, P. (May, 1991). Who killed the nursing care plan? *American Journal of Nursing* 91(5):35–39.

BULECHEK, G., and McCLOSKEY, J. (June, 1992). Defining and validating nursing interventions. *Nursing Clinics of North America* 27(2):289–299.

CARPENITO, L. (1991). *Nursing Care Plans and Documentation.* Philadelphia, Lippincott.

CARROLL-JOHNSON, R.M., (Ed.). (1991). *Classification of Nursing Diagnoses: Proceedings of the Eighth Conference.* North American Nursing Diagnosis Association, Philadelphia, Lippincott.

CARROLL-JOHNSON, R.M. (Ed.). (1991). *Classification of Nursing Diagnoses: Proceedings of the Ninth Conference.* North American Nursing Diagnosis Association, Philadelphia, Lippincott.

GEISSLER, E. (September/October, 1991). Nursing diagnosis of culturally diverse patients. *International Nursing Review* 38(5):150–152.

GIULIANO, K., and POIRIER, C. (March, 1991). Nursing case management: Critical pathways to desirable outcomes. *Nursing Management* 22(3):52–55.

GOODWIN, D. (February, 1992). Critical pathways in home healthcare. *Journal of Nursing Administration* 22(2):35–40.

GORDON, M. (1982). *Nursing Diagnosis: Process and Application.* New York, McGraw-Hill.

GRANT, J., and KINNEY, M. (October/December, 1991). The need for operational definitions for defining characteristics. *Nursing Diagnosis* 2(4):181–185.

GRANT, J., and KINNEY, M. (January/March, 1992). Using the delphi technique to examine the content validity of nursing diagnoses. *Nursing Diagnosis* 3(1):12–22.

HENDERSON, V. (1978). *The Nature of Nursing.* New York, Macmillan.

HERR, K., and MOBILY, P. (June, 1992). Interventions related to pain. *Nursing Clinics of North America* 27(2):347–369.

HILDMAN, T. (May, 1992). Registered nurses' attitudes toward the nursing process and written/printed nursing care plans. *Journal of Nursing Administration*, 22(5):5–6.

HIRAKI, A. (March, 1992). Tradition, rationality and power in introductory nursing textbooks: A critical hermeneutics study. *Advances in Nursing Science* 14(3):1–12.

JOHNSTON, D., and KAPLAN, M. (February, 1993). Medical progress: pathogenesis and treatment of gallstones. *New England Journal of Medicine* 328(6):412–419.

JOINT COMMISSION ON ACCREDITATION OF HEALTHCARE ORGANIZATIONS (1992). *Accreditation Manual for Hospitals.* Vol. 1, *Standards.* Chicago.

KOZIER, B., ERB, G., and OLIVIERI, R. (1991). *Fundamentals of Nursing: Concepts, Process and Practice* (4th ed.). Menlo Park, CA, Addison-Wesley.

MASLOW, A. (1968). *Toward a Psychology of Being.* New York, Van Nostrand.

MCKENZIE, C.B., TORKELSON, N.G., and HOLT, M.A. (1989). Care and cost: Nursing management improves both. *Nursing Management* 10): 30–34.

MOSHER, C., ET AL. (January, 1992). Upgrading practice with critical pathways. *American Journal of Nursing* 91(1):41–44.

NEIDIG, J., MEGEL, M., and KOEHLER, K. (August, 1992). The critical path: An evaluation of the applicability of nursing case management in the NICU. *Neonatal Network* 11(5):45–52.

NORTH AMERICAN NURSING DIAGNOSIS ASSOCIATION. (1992) *NANDA Nursing Diagnoses: Definitions and Classification 1992–1993.* Philadelphia, North American Nursing Diagnosis Association.

OREM, D.E. (1985). *Nursing: Concepts of Practice.* New York, McGraw-Hill.

PIERSON, M., and IRONS, K. (January/March, 1992). Identification of a cluster of nursing diagnoses for a caregiver support group. *Nursing Diagnosis* 3(1): 36–41.

RITTER, J., ET AL. (March, 1992). Redesigning nursing practice: A case management model for critical care. *Nursing Clinics of North America* 27(1): 119–128.

ROY, SISTER C. (1984). *Introduction to Nursing: An Adaptation Model* (2nd. ed.). Norwalk, CT, Appleton-Century-Crofts.

SIEGEL, S. (1992). Telephone follow-up programs as creative nursing interventions. *Pediatric Nursing* 18(1):86–89.

SMELTZER, S., and BARE, B. (1992). *Brunner and Suddarth's Textbook of Medical Surgical Nursing* (7th ed.). Philadelphia, Lippincott.

SMITH, P., ET AL. (September, 1992). Implementing nurse case management in a community hospital. *MedSurg Nursing* 1(1):47–52.

TITLER, M., ET AL. (April/June, 1991). Classification of nursing interventions for care of the integument. *Nursing Diagnosis* 2(2):45–56.

TRIPP, S., and STACHOWIAK, B. (1989). Nursing diagnosis: Health seeking behaviors (specify). In: Carroll-Johnson, R.M., (Ed.). *Classification of Nursing Diagnoses: Proceedings of the Eighth Conference.* (1989). North American Nursing Diagnosis Association, Philadelphia, Lippincott.

WEBER, G. (October, 1991). Making nursing diagnosis work for you and your client. *Nursing and Health Care* 12(8):424–430.

WOOD, R., BAILEY, N., and TILKEMEIER, D. (July, 1992). Managed care: The missing link in quality improvement. *Journal of Nursing Care Quality* 6(4): 55–65.

ZANDER, K. (January, 1988). Managed care within acute care settings: Design and implementation via nursing case management. *Health Care Supervisor* 6(2):27–43.

ZANDER, K. (May, 1988). Nursing case management: Strategic management of cost and quality outcomes. *Journal of Nursing Administration* 18(5):23–30.

ZANDER, K. (September, 1988). Nursing case management. *Nursing Clinics of North America* 23(3):503–520.

ZANDER, K. (Fall, 1991). CareMaps®: The core of cost/quality care. *The New Definition.* 6(3):30–32.

ZANDER, K. (1992). Critical pathways. In: Melum, M., and Sinioris, M. *Total Quality Management.* Chapter 9 (305–314). American Hospital Association, Chicago.

ZANDER, K. (Winter, 1992). Physicians, CareMaps®, and collaboration. *The New Definition.* 7(1):33–36.

ZANDER, K. (May/June, 1992). Focusing on patient outcomes: Case management in the 90s. *Dimensions of Critical Care Nursing* 11(3):127–129.

ZANDER, K. (Fall, 1992). Quantifying, managing and improving quality. *The New Definition.* 7(4):1–4.

Sample Nursing Care Plans

STANDARD PLANS OF CARE

NURSING CARE PLAN #1. MIDDLE ADULT

Lyman, John
66550250
Dr. Burns/Snyder
Room 231 55 yrs

NURSING ASSESSMENT

(Data Collection Format based on the Functional Health Patterns developed by Gordon, 1982)

General Information

Information given by: client

Name: Mr. John Lyman

Age: 55 yrs Sex: male Race: Caucasian

Admission date/time: 7/6/94; 2100 hours

Admitting medical diagnosis: "possible heart attack"

Arrived on unit by: wheelchair   from: home

NURSING CARE PLAN #1 (CONT.)

Accompanied by: daughter

Admitting Weight/VS: T. 99.0, P. 96, R. 28, BP 120/70; 188 lbs, 5'11'

Allergies: no known allergies

Medications: no prescription meds

Health Perception–Health Management

Client's Perception of Reason for Admission: severe pain in middle of chest, upper abdomen region; "The doctor thinks I might have had a heart attack"; "I've never had anything like this before."

How has problem been managed by client at home? "I sat down and tried to relax, then I lay down but nothing helped; the chest pain just kept getting worse so I called the doctor and she said to come right in."

Nutritional-Metabolic Pattern

states he is about 15 lbs overweight; eats 2–3 meals a day, often skips breakfast; cooks for himself but eats out frequently; reports alcohol consumption of 2–3 drinks/week

SKIN: mucous membranes pink; good skin turgor; diaphoretic, pale

LAST INTAKE: at 6 P.M. was a pizza; denies any nausea on admission

FOOD ALLERGIES: none

Elimination Pattern

BOWEL: last BM on 7/6; usual pattern qd; denies taking laxatives/softeners; bowel sounds present in all 4 quadrants

URINARY: denies any changes in urinary elimination patterns: no difficulty initiating; voids in large amounts, no burning; last voiding on admission to hospital—states it was normal large amount

EDEMA: no edema noted in ankles or fingers; denies any problem with edema; ring is not tight

MIDDLE ADULT (CONT.)

Activity-Exercise Pattern

no physical limitations; reports going to the health club 2–3 times a week for weight machines and occasional racquetball games; no daily exercise program

RESPIRATORY: reports slight dyspnea; some diaphoresis noted; respirations nonlabored but slightly deeper and more rapid than normal; lung sounds clear; no cyanosis noted on admission; smokes 2 packs/day; reports he has tried to quit twice but he really enjoys smoking and he lives alone so no one complains

CARDIAC: normal BP 150/90; 120/70 on admission; pulse rapid, strong radial pulse, 96/min and irregular; reports feeling occasional palpitations for last hour; monitor shows normal sinus rhythm, occasional PVC's (1–4/min) over 15 minutes since admission

Sleep-Rest Pattern

6 hours a night is normal pattern; denies use of sleeping medications

Cognitive-Perceptual Pattern

PAIN: states he was watching TV when the pain started in the midchest area; described as viselike and radiated down left arm; "pain got worse and worse over about an hour"; rated as "8" on 1–10 scale

ANALGESICS: states he has taken nothing for pain but really needs something now

SENSES: denies any hearing, speech, or visual problems; states he probably needs glasses because things are getting blurry up as close as he used to hold them; denies any changes in sensation, no numbness of fingers/toes

ORIENTATION: oriented to time, place, and person; states he feels "just awful" and is afraid he is going to die

Self-Perception–Self-Concept Pattern

reports being afraid of dying or being a burden to his family; "my father died of a heart attack in his 50s" and "I have had high blood pressure and an elevated cholesterol for 3 years that I know of"; three married daughters; one lives in town and brought him in; divorced 4 years ago from his wife of 25 years; lives alone and states he is very independent; "couldn't live with my daughters and have them take care of me"; reports he works hard and long

NURSING CARE PLAN #1 (CONT.)

hours as a financial advisor; "my daughters have been after me to take it easier and take some time off but I just never seem to find the time."

Role-Relationship Pattern

lives alone since divorce 4 years ago; ex-wife out of state and does not want her notified of his condition; three married daughters; visits the one in town every few weeks and occasionally babysits his grandchildren

Sexuality-Reproductive Pattern

vasectomy 1969; reports no problems with sexual part of his life; "I've kind of been on hold since the divorce"; "I suppose I won't have to worry about that anymore though; if this is a heart attack I know sex is out for me."

Coping–Stress Tolerance Pattern

"I guess I am under a lot of stress at work; the stock market is hard to predict but my clients expect me to always make a profit; sometimes I feel like everyone is pulling on me to do things for them"; "I'm going to have to make a few phone calls to work, how do I get an outside line?"

Value-Belief Pattern

Catholic; attends church every week; reports he would like to see his priest if he gets worse

Priority Nursing Diagnoses	Outcomes
1. Fear related to possible myocardial infarction and risk of dying as manifested by own statements, elevated pulse	Reduction in fear reported; identification of methods of coping with/reducing fear of MI/dying/reoccurance by disch. ◦ statement of feeling less fearful in 1 hour ◦ states understanding of tests, treatments prior to implementing ◦ states understanding of risk factors in life-style and changes needed to reduce risk by discharge

MIDDLE ADULT (CONT.)

Priority Nursing Diagnoses	Outcomes
2. Pain related to possible myocardial hypoxia as manifested by rating pain an "8," elevated pulse and diaphoresis	Report of negligible pain by discharge ○ pain reported at a level of 3 or less within the next hour with the use of IV morphine ○ pain maintained at a level of 3 or less during the next 48 hours with analgesics
3. High risk for decreased cardiac output related to inadequate pumping of the heart secondary to possible MI (myocardial infarction)	Maintains adequate tissue perfusion during hospitalization ○ maintains clear lung sounds during next 48 hours ○ presence of strong peripheral pulses during next 48 hours ○ maintains heart rate between 70–100 with no cyanosis while hospitalized

Nursing Interventions	Rationale
1. a. Assess understanding and teach prn before tests, tx., interventions.	a. Provides baseline data from which to teach; begin at learner's level of understanding; knowing what to expect decreases fear
b. Offer opportunity to share fears, concerns q4h × 24h; reassure realistically; point out positive sign of status/ functioning.	b. Identifying and discussing fears gives nurse a chance to understand and support without giving false reassurance; focus on positive gives encouragement and hope.
c. Encourage daughter to stay.	c. Presence of support people can decrease fear; increase feelings of safety/security.
d. Have client/family write down their questions for the doctor or nurse.	d. Unanswered questions/ confusion can cause concern; clients often forget to ask questions when MD or nurse in room.
e. Orient to room; all equipment.	e. Unfamiliar environment can cause anxiety/fear.

NURSING CARE PLAN #1 (CONT.)

Nursing Interventions	*Rationale*
f. Offer to contact hospital chaplain anytime client desires.	f. Meeting spiritual needs can decrease anxiety and give hope; opportunity to express concerns.
g. Assign consistent nursing personnel whenever possible: Adams, Grahm, Tran.	g. Development of trusting therapeutic relationship decreases fear.
h. Involve client in planning own care; explain how he can maximize medical and nursing treatment to promote recovery.	h. Gives client sense of control which can decrease fear; promotes cooperation with treatments
i. When physical status stabilizes: ◦ assess knowledge of heart disease and risk factors in his life ◦ provide information as needed ◦ work with client on problem-solving ways to reduce risk factors and attain maximum recovery ◦ discuss possibility of family conference involving daughters, doctor, nurses for discussion of life-style changes; medical management of condition; abilities, limitations, schedule for resumption of activities and work responsibilities.	i. Readiness to learn life-style changes begins with recovery phase of illness; input and support from all involved result in more realistic plan, increased commitment to plan.
2. a. Assess knowledge of reason for pain and assessments; explain as needed to client/family	a. Teaching begins at the learner's level of understanding to be most effective; understanding cause of pain makes tx. more understandable.
b. Assess vital signs and pain; begin morphine IV per doctor's order ◦ respirations, pulse and BP qh	b. Provides baseline data from which response to treatment is judged ◦ morphine can depress respirations

MIDDLE ADULT (CONT.)

Nursing Interventions	Rationale

◦ level of consciousness qh
  ◦ notify MD if r>14, BP>100/70
  ◦ assess and reassure during first 15 min of morphine administration
  ◦ side rail up during administration
	◦ morphine causes vasodilation and possible hypotensive response
	◦ morphine can cause euphoric state; dizziness or fainting can occur if client tries to stand

c. Oxygen per doctor's order; assess concentration, response q 1h	c. Morphine may depress respirations; increasing amount of oxygen to heart tissue will help reduce pain.
d. Position in Semi-Fowler's position (head or bed up at 45 degrees).	d. Generally more comfortable position if SOB; lowers diaphragm and increases lung expansion
e. Explain and implement bed rest order; place urinal, phone, water within reach.	e. Decreases work load on heart and oxygen requirements; may decrease pain
f. Environmental management to promote rest	f. Noisy, bright room with many people talking and doing things interferes with ability to rest and produces added stress/anxiety.
g. Offer techniques to promote relaxation/pain management.	g. Decreased muscle tension reduces oxygen needs of muscles; distraction, imagery can reduce perception of pain and promote rest.

3. a. Assess per doctor's order and report significant changes to physician in areas of:
  ◦ vital signs q1h
  ◦ urine volume q2h or q voiding
  ◦ skin temp/peripheral pulses
  ◦ lung sounds
  ◦ regularity of heartbeat
	a. Assessment data provides baseline for comparison of changes which may indicate changing condition and need for adjustment of nursing and medical treatment plan;
	—decreased urine output may indicate inadequate blood flow to kidney; dehydration
	◦ deterioration in pumping action of heart can lead to dropping BP, increased or decreased heart rate, increase

NURSING CARE PLAN #1 (CONT.)

Nursing Interventions	*Rationale*
	in PVCs; cold pale skin and weak or absent pulses in extremities; buildup of fluid in lungs with moist breath sounds developing
b. Oxygen per doctor's order; assess concentration, response q1h (explain "no smoking" rule).	b. Increased oxygen content of inspired air provides more oxygen to all body tissues; oxygen promotes burning, and smoking could cause a fire.
c. Assist with position changes q2h (head of bed up at 45 degrees).	c. Alternating pressure areas will promote adequate circulation and oxygenation of weight-bearing body tissues.
d. Explain and implement bed rest order, place urinal, phone, water within reach.	d. Decreases work load on heart and improves circulation to legs
e. Accurate intake-output recordings and daily weights	e. Dehydration can decrease the circulating blood volume resulting in decreased perfusion of periphery; excess fluid can cause accumulation in the lungs; maintenance of normal weight reflects adequate hydration and no fluid retention.

NURSING CARE PLAN #1. MIDDLE ADULT

(demonstrates individualization of pretyped form for dx of "Pain")

Lyman, John
66550250
Dr. Burns/Snyder
Room 231   55 yrs

Nursing Diagnosis Standard Care Plan: Pain

Pain related to *myocardial hypoxia 7/6/94*

("A state in which an individual experiences and reports the presence of severe discomfort or an uncomfortable sensation," NANDA, 1992).

Client Characteristics: *pain rated as "8" on admission, P96, R28, diaphoretic*

Client Goals/Outcome Standards:

✓ Verbalization that pain has been eliminated or decreased to a level of ___*3*___ on a scale of 1–10 by *1 hr with use of IV morphine drip*
during *next 48 hrs c̄ analgesics*

___ Evaluation: _____

NA Reduction of agitated/restless behavior by _____ .
___ Evaluation: _____

✓ Reduction in values of vital signs, Ⓟ Ⓡ BP, toward normal range by __*4 hrs*__.
___ Evaluation: _____

Other: *Report of negligible pain by discharge c̄ no analgesics*
___ Evaluation: _____

Nursing Intervention Standards:

✓ 1. Assess pain and related factors.
  a. intensity (1–10) *8 on adm   2100 hrs   7/6*
  b. duration *1 hr while at home*
  c. character (sharp, dull, shooting, burning) *viselike; radiates L arm*
  d. location *midchest & down L arm*
  e. precipitated by *unknown; no precipitating exercise/activity*

✓ 2. Assess for effectiveness of previous pain relief interventions
  a. previous medication (drug, dose, route, effectiveness on 1–10)
     denies any
  b. other helpful measures: *none; sitting & lying at home not helpful.*

NURSING CARE PLAN #1 (CONT.)

✓ 3. Offer _IV morphine sulfate_ (analgesic ordered by MD) _continuous drip_ prn.

_NA_ 4. Encourage use of analgesics before _____
      (pain precipitating activity) at _____ A.M./P.M. or _____

✓ 5. Offer relaxation techniques: slow relaxed breathing _✓; relaxation_
music _____ heat _____
      backrub _✓ q2h_ other _____

✓ 6. Assist with repositioning (specify) _Semi-Fowlers_ q _2 hrs_

✓ 7. Encourage use of distracting stimuli: radio, TV, effleurage, other:
      imagery; quiet environment

Developed by _L. Atkinson R.N._ date: _7/6/94_

Evaluated by _____ date: _____

Reviewed/Updated by _____ date: _____

NURSING CARE PLAN #2. SENIOR ADULT

Morgan, Fred
89645412
Dr. Sharp/Johnson
Room 109   78 years

NURSING ASSESSMENT

(Data Collection Format based on Human Response Patterns described by NANDA, 1992)

General Information

Information given by: client and son

Name: Mr. Fred Morgan   Age: 78 yrs   Sex: male   Race: Caucasian

Admission date/time: 12/1/94; 2 P.M.

Admitting medical diagnosis: unable/unwilling to care for self at home; weight loss; mild hypertension history

Arrived on unit by: wheelchair   from: home

Accompanied by: son

Admitting Weight/VS: T. 97.0, P. 90, R. 20, BP 140/88; 154 lbs, 6'1"

Client's Perception of Reason for Admission: "I don't need to be here. I'm

SENIOR ADULT (CONT.)

just tired. I was fine when my wife was alive but now I don't get out much or do anything. My son's worried I don't eat."

How had problem been managed by client at home? son visits every few weeks but says father is getting worse, isolated, losing weight

Allergies: no known allergies

Medications: "something for my blood pressure" (Inderal)

Exchanging

NUTRITION: wears dentures, states they do not hurt; lips are pink but dry; poor skin turgor; appears gaunt, thin; reports normal smell but decreased taste to food; reports poor appetite; cooks for self; "Food just doesn't taste good any more"; son states father does not eat, won't shop for groceries; has lost 11 lbs in the last 2 months

ELIMINATION: continent of bowel and bladder; denies taking laxatives; states normal pattern q.d.; denies trouble initiating or maintaining urination; voids large amounts several times a day

CIRCULATION: heart rate 90 and regular; strong pulses; BP 140/88 on admission; son states it used to be higher and father put on medication several years ago; feet and hands pale, cool

OXYGENATION: breath sounds clear; rate 20/minute; nonlabored; denies smoking; son says he quit 15 years ago; denies any difficulty breathing; son says lately his father tires easily and breathes harder with activity

PHYSICAL INTEGRITY: skin intact, dry; mucous membranes intact, no open sores; son states father was not bathing, shaving, or doing personal hygiene; nails dirty

Communication

initiates no conversation; responds only to direct questions; denies any hearing problem; speech not impaired

Relating

SOCIALIZATION: son states father used to be outgoing and was active with his wife in church and around the house; son states father has progressively with-

NURSING CARE PLAN #2 (CONT.)

drawn from contact and communication with friends/family since wife's death 6 months ago

ROLE: son states father was a carpenter but remained active with projects after retirement but now he doesn't do anything; doesn't call family or relate to grandchildren when visiting; patient states "I've got nothing to do; no point in doing anything anymore" denies having any close friends, "They are all dead or put away"; says son busy with his own life and doesn't have time for him (son lives out of town, 1 hour away; client's only child)

Valuing

states he used to go to church with his wife every Sunday but he did it for her so now there's no point going

Choosing

COPING: "I just don't care any more"; reports thinking about wife frequently. Son says his father is having trouble making even simple decisions so leaves bills, shopping, cooking, and so on unattended

Moving

MOBILITY–ACTIVITY: son reports father tires more easily since he has lost weight, "stopped caring about himself"; no physical limitations; no activities except watching TV

REST–SLEEP: client states tired all the time; can't sleep, wakes up 2–3 times/ night; naps frequently; son states he is always sleeping in chair when he visits

ACTIVITIES OF DAILY LIVING: son states he thinks father is able to live alone and manage for himself but just doesn't care anymore

Perceiving

SELF-CONCEPT: states he is "useless"; feels "helpless without his wife"; "no good to anyone any more"

SENSORY–PERCEPTION: no changed sensations; wears bifocals; states he hears well

Knowing/Thought Processes

no evidence of altered thought processes; sentences logical, appropriate responses; oriented to time, place, and person

SENIOR ADULT (CONT.)

Feeling

COMFORT: denies any pain; "stiff sometimes"

EMOTIONAL STATE/INTEGRITY: crying occasionally during assessment; "I can't understand why she had to die. I wish it had been me. Its hard to be the one left." "I want to be with her again." Denies feeling suicidal, "I wouldn't do that."

Priority Nursing Diagnoses	*Outcomes*
1. Altered nutrition: less than body requirements related to lack of interest in food as manifested by 11 lb. weight loss over last 2 months.	1. Weight will stabilize at his previous level of 165 lbs. within 3 months. Evaluate 5/1 ∘ weight gain of 3 lbs at the end of 2 weeks. Evaluate 2/15 ∘ report of appetite returning during the next week. Evaluate on 2/8
2. Sleep pattern disturbance related to loss of wife, altered daytime activity pattern, frequent naps as evidenced by statements of inability to get to sleep, wakening 2–3 times per night, being tired all the time.	2. Sleeping 6 hours through the night during stay in nursing home.
3. Dysfunctional grieving related to death of spouse as manifested by report of constantly thinking about his wife, crying, self-imposed social isolation, physical neglect of self.	3. Reestablishes previous level of self-care, productivity, social contacts by 3/1 ∘ expresses feelings related to loss of spouse within 1 week ∘ identifies losses/changes in his life because of wife's death by 2nd week ∘ identifies self-destructive or punishing behavior in self by 2 weeks ∘ independently reestablishes previous level of personal grooming by 4 weeks

NURSING CARE PLAN #2 (CONT.)

Priority Nursing Diagnoses	Outcomes
4. Low self-esteem: situational, related to loss of spouse and husband role as manifested by statements of helplessness, uselessness, inability to do anything productive.	4. Evaluate self as needed and competent by 3 months ◦ one positive statement of self-worth within 48 hours ◦ begins work on one carpentry project by 2 weeks
5. High risk for violence: self-directed related to negative self-esteem and depression as manifested by statements of wanting to be with dead wife, wishing it had been him that died.	5. Client will deny suicidal plans or ideas throughout stay in nursing home. Evaluate Fridays of each week.

Nursing Interventions	Rationale
1. a. Observe, record, and report I & O.	1. a.b. Monitor client's progress/ evaluate effectiveness of plan.
b. Weigh q A.M.	
c. Assess food preferences.	c. Taking into account client's likes/dislikes may stimulate appetite.
d. Assist client in filling out daily menu.	d. Involve client in plan to increase cooperation. Ensure nutritionally balanced meal.
e. Consult with physician and dietitian regarding between-meal snacks, high calorie and high protein food supplements, possible vitamin supplements.	e. Meet nutritional needs of client.
f. Assist client with hygiene before meals.	f. Increase psychological and physical readiness to eat.
g. Encourage client to sit with others in the dining room @ mealtimes.	g. Normal eating situation tends to stimulate appetite.
2. a. Obtain a sleep history on pattern prior to death of wife and changes since death.	2. a. Provides baseline data from which to assess activities that promote or interfere with sleep

SENIOR ADULT (CONT.)

Nursing Interventions	Rationale
b. Assess for factors in nursing home environment that might interfere with sleep and minimize if possible.	b. Noise, heat, cold, too hard or soft a bed, roommates, lights, can all interfere with sleep.
c. Increase daytime activity ○ dining room for meals ○ shower/bath daily; patient's choice ○ walks on grounds/in building for 10–15 minutes QID ○ encourage participation in group exercise sessions/activities	c. Promotes normal circadian rhythm
d. Offer back rub at HS.	d. Backrubs help to relax muscles and provide the client time to talk about any concerns; relaxation and decreased anxiety facilitate sleep.
e. Encourage good sleep hygiene ○ no caffeine after noon meal ○ limit cigarette smoking ○ offer light snack before bed ○ help to follow usual routine for hygiene, time to retire	e. ○ caffeine is a stimulant ○ nicotine can stimulate CNS ○ foods high in protein and L-tryptophan (milk) promote sleep ○ normal habits from home are associated with a good sleeping pattern
3. a. Assess the existence, extent and impact of unresolved losses through use of open-ended and direct questions.	3. a. Must assess types of unresolved losses and importance to client in order to fully implement plan (Note: elderly frequently have multiple unresolved losses).
b. Encourage client to verbalize feelings regarding losses.	b.c. Increase data base; assist client in developing an awareness of predominant feelings.

NURSING CARE PLAN #2 (CONT.)

Nursing Interventions	*Rationale*
c. Share own observations of client's behavior and seek clarification/confirmation.	
d. Spend 10 min sitting c̄ client b.i.d.; use touch as appropriate; remain c̄ client despite lack of ability to verbalize.	d. Build rapport, develop trust. Convey unconditional acceptance so client is free to express feelings.
e. Look over the daily activity calendar c̄ the client and leave a copy in his room; specifically suggest choosing one activity.	e. Involve client to improve cooperation. Individualize plan to ensure its likelihood of success. Decrease isolation.
f. Encourage client to sit c̄ others in the dining room @ meal times.	f.g. Gradually "repeople" client's life; supply opportunities for development of meaningful interpersonal relationships s̄ overwhelming him. Reinforce sense of belonging.
g. Introduce cient to other residents on the units.	
4. a. Assess client's interests through use of open-ended and direct questions.	4. a. Necessary data to guide plan.
b. Encourage client to verbalize about himself, especially his present feelings.	b. Continue assessment. Convey acceptance of client. Increase client awareness of feelings.
c. Continue nursing actions 3.c. and 3.d.	c. Same as 3.c. and 3.d.
d. Maximize choices client can make.	d.e.f. Rebuild self-esteem.
e. Assist c̄ grooming as needed.	
f. Give merited praise and recognition based on specific, accurate observation.	

SENIOR ADULT (CONT.)

Nursing Interventions	Rationale
g. Occupational therapy referral for projects, needs of facility in carpentry.	g. Projects useful to facility in field of expertise reinforce usefulness, positive self-worth.
5. a. Be direct in asking client if he is presently suicidal.	5. a. Determine immediate need for intervention.
b. Make verbal agreement c̄ client that he will notify nursing staff if feeling out of control or suicidal.	b. Involve client in plan to ensure its success.
c. Move client to room closer to nurse's station if feeling suicidal.	c. Increase nurse's accessibility to client and increase opportunities for observation.
d. Increase frequency of room checks.	d. Prevent, interfere with, or interrupt any self-destructive behavior.
e. Monitor client behavior; observe especially for changes in mood/or levels of energy (be aware of greater risk following these changes).	e. Provide data c̄ which to evaluate suicide potential; changes may signal increased suicide risk.
f. Alert all staff regarding client's suicidal potential.	f. Provide safety and security for client.
g. Spend 10 min. sitting c̄ client b.i.d.; use touch as appropriate; remain c̄ client despite lack of verbalization.	g. Build rapport, develop trust. Convey unconditional acceptance so client is free to express feelings.
h. Permit verbalization of suicidal feelings, do not ignore them or argue c̄ client about them.	h. Establish trust. Recognize importance of intent.
i. Carefully document client behavior and nursing actions.	i. Ensure consistency of care.

NURSING CARE PLAN #2. SENIOR ADULT

(demonstrates individualization of pretyped form for **dx** of "Altered Nutrition")

Morgan, Fred
89645412
Dr. Sharp/Johnson
Room 109   78 yrs

Nursing Diagnosis Standard Care Plan: Altered Nutrition

Altered Nutrition: less than body requirements related to *lack of* _____

interest in food; progressively worse since wife's death _____

("The state in which an individual experiences an intake of nutrients insufficient to meet metabolic needs," NANDA, 1992)

Client Characteristics: *weight loss of 11 lbs in last 2 months; appears gaunt,*

dry skin, poor turgor, states "Food just doesn't taste good anymore" _____

_____

Client Goals/Outcome Standards:

NA Maintains current weight by _____ for _____
    Evaluation: _____

NA Tolerates diet of _____ by _____
    Evaluation: _____

✓ Gains *3 lbs* _____ each day/week/month *every 2 wks* by *12/15*
    Evaluation: _____

✓ Consumes _____ calories/day or *50% or more* % of meals
    by *12/3* _____
    Evaluation: _____

✓ Identifies factors contributing to inadequate intake by *12/5*
Evaluation: _____

✓ Client demonstrates ability to (plan)(prepare) *2000 calorie*
    diet to meet needs by *time of discharge if able to leave nursing home*
    Evaluation: _____

✓ Reports good appetite by *12/8* _____
    Evaluation: _____

✓ Regains lost weight of _____ *11* _____ lbs by *3/1/95* _____ ; maintains
    target weight of *165 or ↑* for *duration of stay in nursing home*
____ Evaluation: _____

SENIOR ADULT (CONT.)

Other: _____

    Evaluation: _____

Nursing Intervention Standards:
1. Assess current dietary intake and related factors.
   a. meals/snacks per day *snacks when hungry; eats Bkf & small supper*
   b. types of foods eaten *sandwiches, cereal, toast*
   c. changes in eating patterns *wife used to cook all meals -B,L,D*
   d. factors interfering with adequate intake (physical)(psychological), finan-
      cial, (educational) *↓ appetite; ↓ sense of taste, no groceries*
      in home, doesn't like to shop or cook for self
   e. favorite foods/fluids *wife's cooking; meat & potatoes*
   f. help needed with eating *none; enc. to eat*
2. Assist with meals by *enc. out of bed & to dining room; enc. to eat at least*
   1/2 of each food on tray; praise
3. Problem solve with client/family on ways to reduce factors interfering with
   adequate diet.
   Discharge planning should include senior meals program delivered to home
   _____
4. Referral to (dietary) social service/public health nurse/other *physician*
   for any diet restrictions related to hypertension
5. Record I&O; encourage (client)/family participation in recording.
6. Offer opportunity for (client)/family to talk about reasons for not eating
   qd at H.S.
7. Encourage smaller meals; *choc. shake* in between snacks; favorite foods
8. Adapt environmental factors to promote appetite/eating *open curtains;*
   time for cleaning dentures & out of bed b/4 meals
9. Weigh: *qd & record*
10. Good oral hygiene before and after meals, self ✓ *enc.* assist _____
11. Promote socialization during meals by: *intro to other residents in dining room.*
12. Other interventions: *Discuss relationship between grief & depression; effect on*
    appetite; food consumption

Developed by *L. Atkinson R.N. 12/1/94*

Index